water

PURE THERAPY

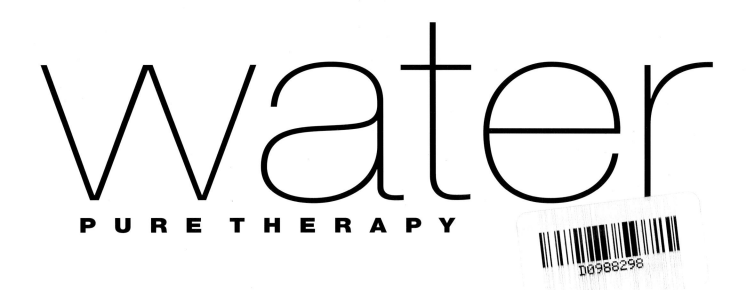

ALICE KAVOUNAS

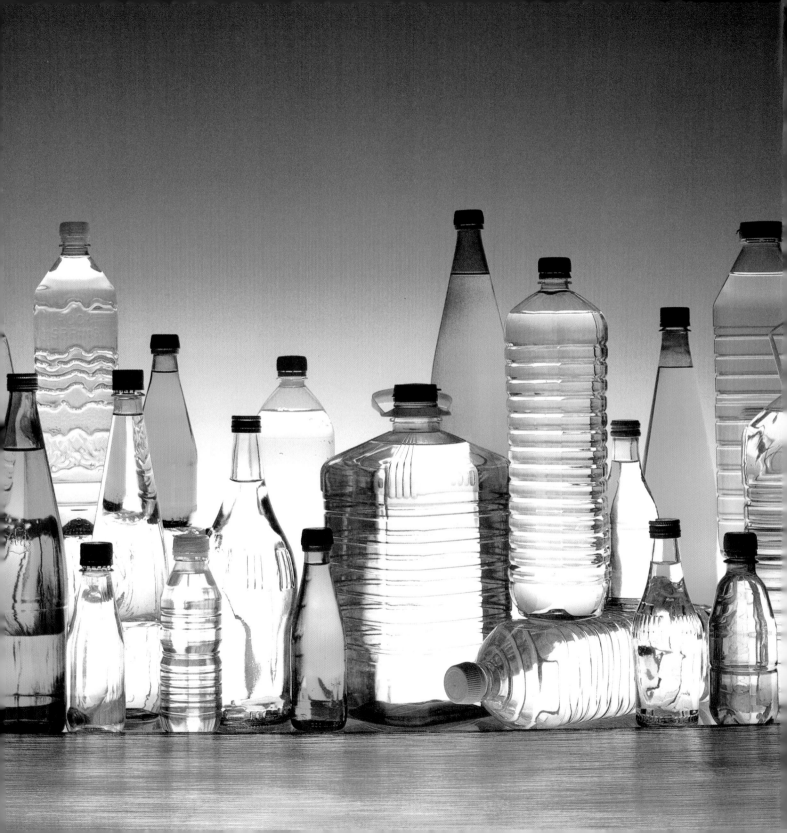

water

PURE THERAPY

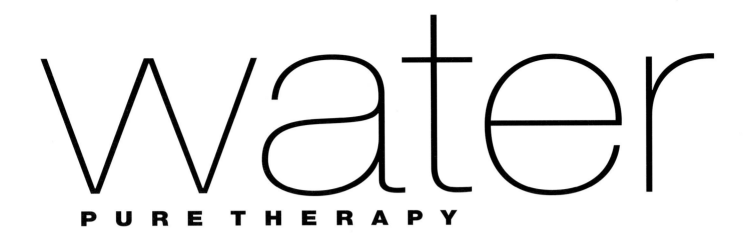

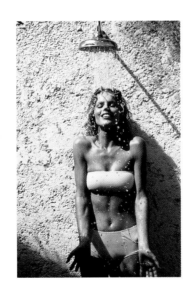

BY ALICE KAVOUNAS

This book is dedicated to David Evans

First published in Great Britain in 2000 by
Kyle Cathie Limited
122 Arlington Road
London NW1 7HP
general.enquiries@kyle-cathie.com

ISBN 1 85626 352 5

Text © 2000 Alice Kavounas
Photography © 2000 Laura Hodgson, except for those listed on page 160.

Design: XAB
Project Editors: Kirsten Abbott/Helen Woodhall
Editorial Assistant: Georgina Burns

Alice Kavounas is hereby identified as the author of this work in accordance with Section 77 of the Copyright, Designs and Patents Act 1988

A CIP catalogue record for this title is available from the British Library

Colour separations by Colourscan, Singapore
Printed and bound in Singapore by Kyodo Printing Co.

contents

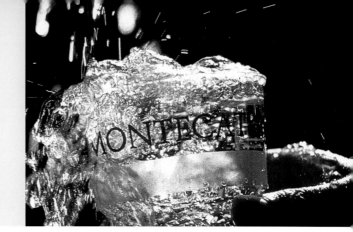

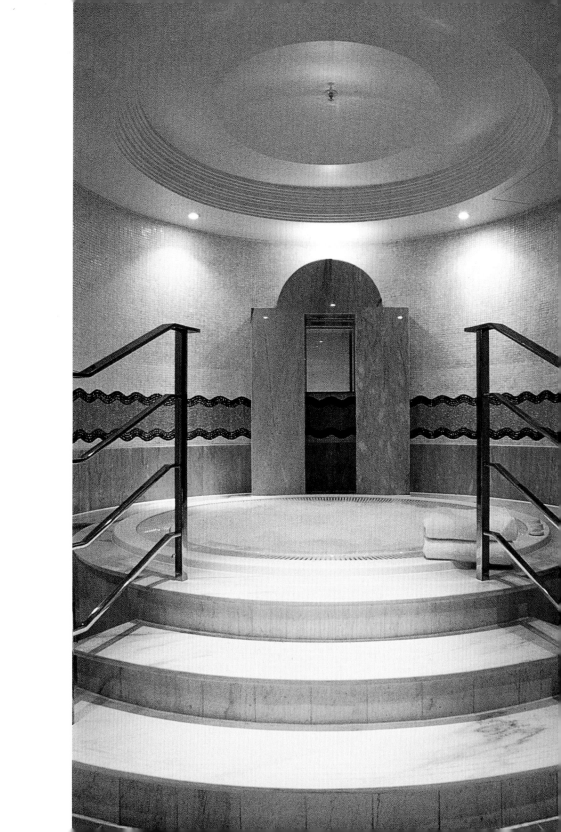

introduction

The sea is pounding the Cornish coast, the January gales are whipping 'round the house, the fat-budded camellias are coming into flower and the palm trees in our coastal garden are thriving. Here on this wild, yet mild peninsula, we're rich in life's key resource.

Water. As schoolchildren, we learn that the human body is about 70% water.

I still pinch and pummel my all too solid flesh and bone and think, how can we be made mostly of water? But it's true. Moreover, every five to ten days we need to replace it to stay alive and functioning. But it wasn't scientific curiosity that originally drew me to this subject. And although I was born under the sign of Cancer, live surrounded by water, and come from a Greek heritage, that country synonymous with the sea, the idea for this book was sparked by a migraine. . .

Like millions of others, I've long been plagued by migraines. Following a particularly bad run of them, I was recommended to David Evans, a gifted cranial osteopath. His skill involves the gentle manipulation of the cranial hemispheres and of the soft tissue. Like all organs, these 'float' in an aqueous solution and shifts of even fractions of a millimetre can affect your well-being. But David insisted that osteopathy alone would not solve my problem – I was dehydrated which was exacerbating the pain. Water was central to his treatment.

Initially, drinking eight glasses of water a day sounds quite boring and difficult. Strangely, the more I drank, the thirstier I became. I began to feel lighter, my eyes and skin looked clearer, my hair seemed to thicken again. Most important of all, my migraines diminished. Now, drinking eight glasses is as natural as breathing. Without it, I feel like a dog in a hot car: dehydrated.

Water is vital therapy in every form – liquid, ice, and steam – but it must be pure. What does that mean? I decided I needed to know much more. After all, millions of us are now bottled-water babies because of our concern for the deteriorating taste and quality of tap water, fear of unknown contaminants. Only now that I've researched the subject do I know what natural mineral water means, whether 'table', or 'spring water' is any healthier than what emerges from the tap.

Soon I found myself wondering not just about watering your body, but about the need to water your soul. Bathing as ritual, as soul-therapy. This book has taken me on a wonderful pilgrimage, leading me to sacred wells just miles from where I live; to holistic spas where women and men find rejuvenation and respite from stressful lives; reminding me time and again of my own cultural origins, and of myriad links with the earliest civilisations. Look, and you will discover your own ways of watering body and soul. More than just a life-giving drink, water is integral to existence, capable of shaping your inner and outer being in extraordinary ways.

WATERING YOUR BODY

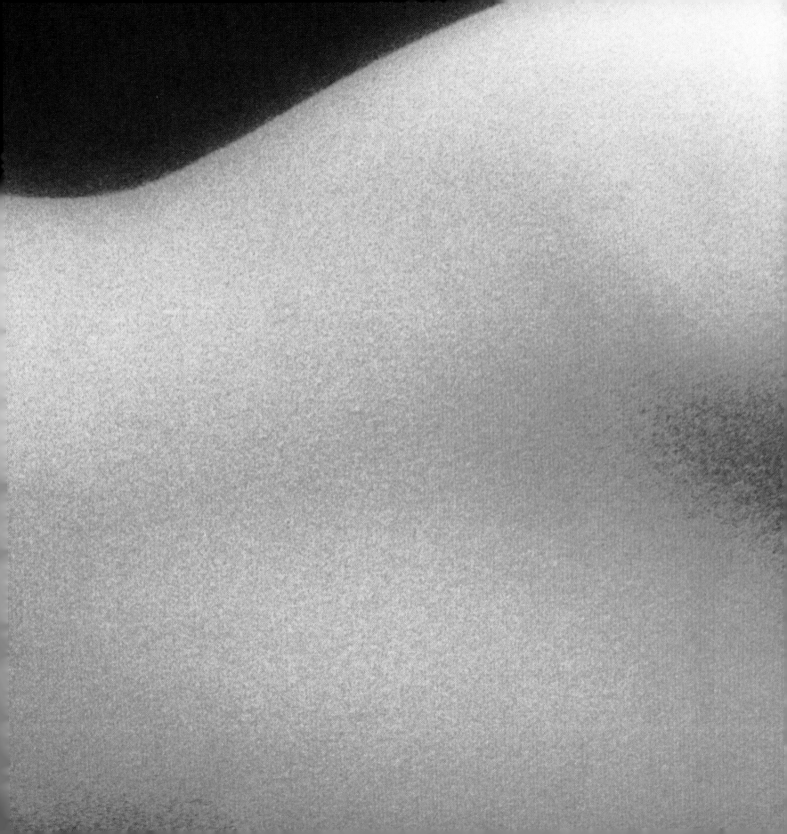

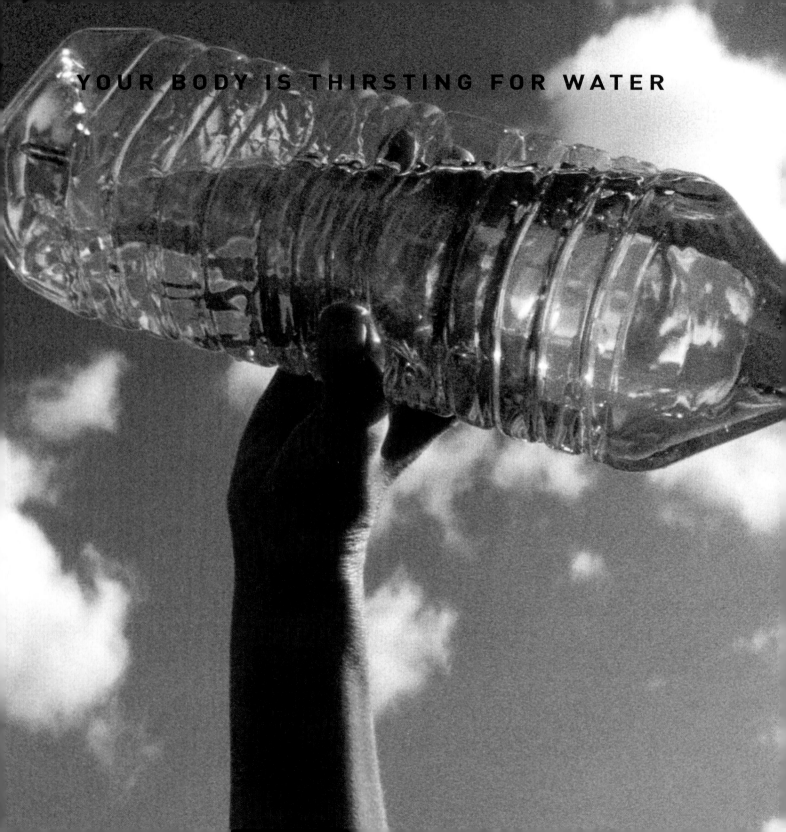

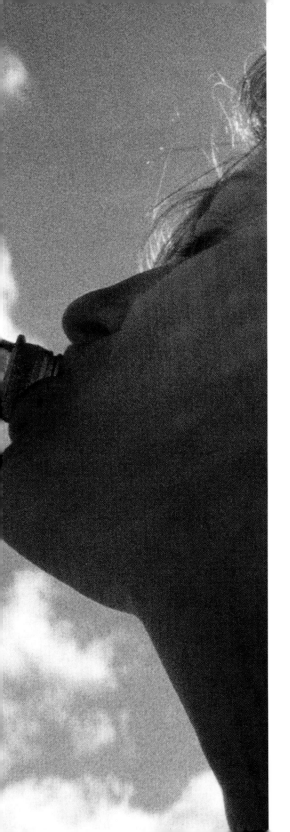

...the word freighted with the greatest weight of longing is *dipsa*, thirst, and in love poems lovers drink the dew from each other's lips, and are refreshed in each other's arms as if dew fell on them.

PATRICIA STORACE
DINNER WITH PERSEPHONE

As children we are amazed to learn that two thirds of our body weight is water. I still pinch and pummel my all-too-solid flesh and bone and think, *impossible*! But all cells contain water (even bone and blood cells), and they are surrounded by it as if by a mini-ocean. Your body needs water to function – not to function better; it needs water to function. Yet it is so easy to forget to drink enough water. Relax. Forgetting is not your fault, as I will explain – along with what to do about it.

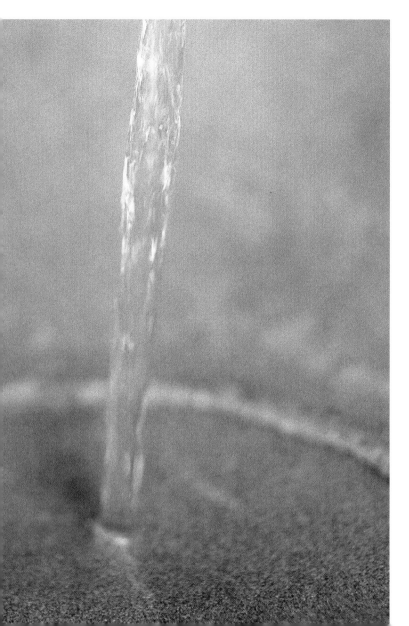

First take a look at the crucial role water plays in the internal workings of your body's day-to-day life. It is not something you probably give much thought to, and I want you to see from the very start of this book why it is that without the pure therapy of water you cannot expect to feel and look healthy and fit.

Medical journalist Dr Jane Clarke, writing on the importance of water in *The Observer Magazine*, believes that water 'is a must for a healthy, energetic body'. You need water to enable your body to keep eliminating toxic substances, to produce digestive enzymes, maintain healthy skin, hair and organs, and to help your body absorb essential vitamins, minerals and natural sugars. Water also regulates your body temperature, cooling you down by evaporating through your skin.

A lack of water can play havoc with your body, however balanced your diet. According to Dr Clarke, even high cholesterol and triglyceride levels 'can be aggravated by lack of water'. Do you have a good, healthy diet with lots of fibre? Great. Now add water to make the most of it! Without enough water in your system, whole grains, pulses, oats, fruits and vegetables 'cannot swell and stimulate the body to produce high-density lipoprotein, aka 'good cholesterol'. HDL picks up low-density lipoprotein – 'bad cholesterol' – and takes it to the gut, where it is excreted.

...even on a cool day your body uses and loses 2 litres (3½ pints) of water.

Water is your body's most important nutrient

Patrick Holford, founder of the Institute for Optimum Nutrition in London and author of *The Optimum Nutrition Bible* calls water 'the forgotten nutrient' in the diet of sportsmen and sportswomen. I would go one further and describe it as the forgotten nutrient in almost everyone's diet. Edmund Burke, Professor of Exercise Science at the University of Colorado, explains: 'Look at your circulation system as if it were an automobile engine. Just as water helps a car run more efficiently by enabling fuel to move through the machinery to the engine, so water delivers oxygen and nutrients through the bloodstream to your muscles.' Muscles, by the way, are 75 per cent water.

You might find this difficult to visualise, but even on a cool day your body uses and loses 2 litres (3½ pints) of water. Water is excreted through your skin and kidneys, and with every exhalation of breath (just breathe onto a mirror). Two litres: ideally, that's what you need to take in every day – not counting water in the foods you eat. But do you? If not, it could it be because you don't *feel* thirsty.

Seeing thirst is simple if you are looking at a drooping flower. Sensing it in yourself is much harder, especially on a cool day when you are just going about your normal round of activities. If you live in the tropics, you are bound to be more thirst-conscious. Otherwise, it seems that only on blazing hot days, when you have been exercising, or perhaps had too much alcohol (or all three together!) does your body 'tell' you that you are dehydrated. A dry mouth, fatigue and flushed skin are all late rather than early warning signs that your body is thirsting for water. Your thirst alarm doesn't alert you when it should, so you could easily be dehydrated, as I was, without realising it. A Gallup survey commissioned by the Natural Mineral Water Information Service in April 1999 revealed that the majority of people in the UK drink less than 1 litre (1¾pints) of water a day, half the amount doctors recommend. In the USA, 80 per cent of the population drinks less water than the recommended daily 2 litres (3½pints).

Scientists are still unravelling the mystery of thirst

Thirst – like hunger, sleep and emotion – is regulated by the brain's hypothalamus. This appears to be sensitive to the salts which exist within that mini-ocean throughout your body. As your water level drops, the salt concentration increases. At last! Off goes your thirst alarm. By this time you could already be starving some of your vital organs, including your brain, of your body's most important nutrient: water. Why is salt the trigger? One explanation is that salt maintains cell structure and cells cannot determine how much water they need, only how much salt. Cells receive those salts through the process of osmosis and water is essential to put the salts in solution.

Water is *the* dynamic element which recharges your body, irrigating and invigorating every vital organ. Stop drinking water and you stagnate – headaches, lethargy, constipation, muscle and joint aches, increased cellulite deposits where toxins accumulate, and, potentially, serious kidney and cardiovascular problems follow from dehydration. You can go without food for weeks, but not without water.

you do not always feel as thirsty as you obviously are. Holford points out: 'During athletic performance thirst sensors are inhibited, so it is easy for athletes to become dehydrated.' Your body, even at times of great need, does not necessarily tell you fast enough that you should top up your water level. According to Holford in *The Optimum Nutrition Bible*, a loss of only 3 per cent of your body's water content causes a 10 per cent drop in strength and an 8 per cent loss of speed. To avoid dehydration Holford advises you to prepare yourself by

if your body's water supplies are low, it is your skin that suffers

You might be wondering at this point how you have managed to stay alive if you never drink even one glass of water a day. The answer is that foods contain water, which adds to your daily intake. Your body relies on what you are eating and drinking. (Your body cells also produce a small amount of water as a by-product of breathing.) This limited way of attaining water is not ideal. But your body is smart, grabbing water from wherever it can for its most vital functions, leaving other organs to make do with what is left.

Your skin, for example, the body's biggest organ, is a huge reservoir of water but is the last to benefit from it, so if your body's water supplies are low, your skin suffers. (Normally the skin's inner layer (dermis) is made up of 70 per cent water.) Skin tends to become drier with age; also, older people may feel less thirsty. So it is doubly important that as you grow older, you drink more water. Since drinking 2 litres daily my skin has more spring to it; my complexion is clearer.

If you are an active sportsperson, you probably know the dangers of dehydration, but you might not have realised why

drinking a glass of water every fifteen minutes for one to four hours before an event, depending on its length. I include this because it is good advice whether or not you are planning to run a marathon. Before you engage in any physical exercise, prepare for it by drinking enough water to keep yourself hydrated throughout your exercise routine. You will be rewarded with more energy, and be less likely to grab at fizzy drinks or cappuccinos the minute you have finished. (Caffeine, like alcohol, is a diuretic. Both will deplete your stores of water, carrying with them essential vitamins and minerals.)

Pale yellow is good news

Check the colour of your urine. This test may be more accurate than waiting for the sensation of thirst. It is a simple way to tell whether or not you are drinking enough water for your kidneys to excrete wastes and toxins. A very pale yellow is good news. If it is dark, and you urinate infrequently, you could be putting your kidneys under strain. A few days after you have started drinking more water you will notice the colour change.

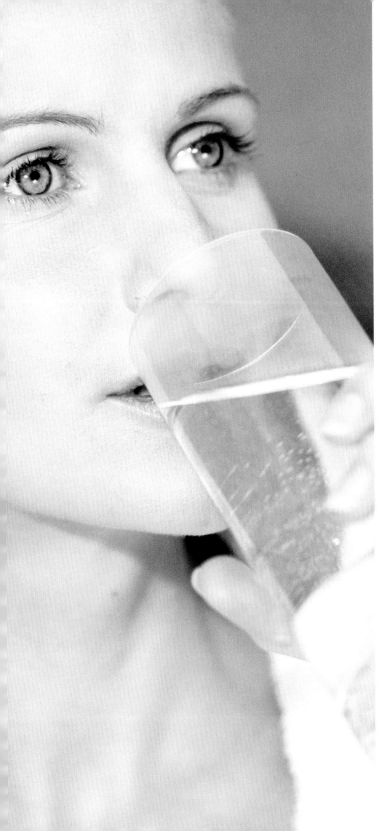

The more water you drink, the thirstier you will feel

I began by saying that even on a cool day your body uses and loses 2 litres (3½ pints) of water, more if you are exercising or if it is hot. Remember, these 2 litres enable your body to function; they do not act as a bonus element to allow you to engage in extraordinary bursts of activity. They are essential for your health and well-being however sedentary or athletic you are.

Just as a plant needs water to survive and stay upright (let alone grow), so you need water on a day-in day-out basis. And, yes, it is strange that your body's thirst alarm does not work more effectively. But here is an even stranger observation: *The more water you drink, the thirstier you will feel*. This has happened not only to me, but to all the people I know who have started to drink more water. They now feel they need to drink that water! Is thirst so different from hunger? If you skip one meal, you feel hungry, but if you go on a fast for a few days, you begin to lose the sensation of hunger. Considering that you have not been drinking water on any consistent basis for years, it is no wonder your body may have buried this thirst sensation.

I never felt thirsty unless I was on a hot beach all day, or if I had (unwisely) consumed an entire bag of crisps. Now my body demands its daily 2 litres no matter what the temperature, no matter what I'm doing that day. And drinking those 2 litres is easy! Don't worry about which water to drink; the pros and cons of tap, filtered, natural mineral and spring waters are covered later in this book. Simply start with one that tastes good to you and follow the step by step plan outlined in the following pages. Before long you will have activated your sleepy thirst alarm and you will be drinking with ease and pleasure the 2 litres of water your body uses and loses each day.

The motivation

'Dehydration lowers blood volume and reduces the flow to muscles and brain. The more dehydrated you become, the more you will feel lethargic, tired and irritable. A headache could be the first sign,' says nutritionist Lyndel Costain of the British Dietetic Association. Costain suggests that the best 'spring clean' you can give your body is a weekend of healthy eating while drinking between 1.5 and 2 litres (2⅔ and 3½ pints) of water a day. A weekend like that is an excellent way to start your programme of water therapy. In fact it is a good way to carry on for the rest of the year. Before I discuss method, however, let's talk motivation, because unless you know why you are doing something, you probably won't keep it up whatever the method.

authority Leslie Kenton, in *10 Steps to a New You*, believes: 'After oxygen water is the most important thing you consume – more important, even, than your foods, although they contain some of the most beneficial water you will ever take into your body.'

I have suffered from severe migraines since I was ten years old. My primary motivation for making sure I drink an adequate amount of water every day is to prevent them. Dehydration is a key factor that brings on my migraines. It was identified by David Evans, DO, a cranial osteopath who believes that dehydration is all too common and a major cause of the body's malfunctioning. It is he who is the inspiration behind this book. Whatever he can accomplish through the manipulation of tissue and bone, he told me in

'Dehydration lowers blood volume and reduces the flow to muscles and brain.

Food fads come and go. Some catch on, some don't. Ditto for diets. Some work, some don't. The starkly simple concept that you should drink at least 2 litres of water each day is central to most diets (but usually overlooked), and it is here to stay. The word 'hydrotherapy' comes from the ancient Greek for water – hydro – and although the term now refers to external water therapy, originally it included taking in the waters as well as taking them lying down. Water was key to a holistic approach to health two thousand years ago, and all this time later a simple drink of water remains vital to your health, fitness and looks. Until you start drinking water, day in, day out, you will not entirely believe it. Health and fitness

an early session, is as nothing compared to what a daily intake of 2 litres of fresh water can do. I began to drink water that day and have felt better ever since. As is the case with many osteopaths, his approach is holistic. He gave me the impetus to take the simple step forward to improve my health – by suggesting water not as a cure-all, but as the main ingredient in a healthier way of life.

I believe strongly that no one thing works on its own to promote good health. I agree with David's holistic approach, and recommend you use water therapy along with whatever other measures you take. Like most ailments, my migraines are caused by several other factors as well as dehydration:

tension and tiredness are two. Just as dehydration is not the only cause, rehydration in and of itself will never be the whole cure. However, drinking enough water every day can act like a healing river through your body, easing and improving a myriad of conditions, making you feel better immediately and over the long term.

As you know from reports in the media, there is usually extensive disagreement over health matters in terms both of causes and cures. Yet everyone agrees about the importance of drinking water. This has motivated me to keep drinking water, even when it occasionally seems inconvenient. From mainstream medical doctors to a wide range of alternative professionals including osteopaths and nutritionists, from sports scientists to your personal trainer (should you be so lucky as to have one) and, if you asked her, probably even your mother – all agree that water holds the key to achieving and maintaining optimum health, which in turn enhances your looks.

Your reasons for beginning to rehydrate your body will be different from mine. For example, which of the following would you like to live without: headaches, constipation, cystitis, lethargy, back pain, water retention, high cholesterol, excess weight?

And which of these would you like to improve: the tone and texture of your skin, your circulation, your digestion, your concentration? As an added bonus, would you like to feel less hungry between meals? Reduce the cellulite around your hips and thighs? Increase your daily levels of energy and vitality?

You can significantly improve one or several of these conditions by drinking 2 litres of water a day. It couldn't be simpler. What are you waiting for?

The method

Question: How many shrinks does it take to change a light bulb? Answer: Only one, but the light bulb has to really, really want to change.

I am assuming you really, really want to feel and look better, and that you are beginning to be convinced by now that water will help you, for whichever combination of reasons I've outlined.

If the prospect of drinking 2 litres of water a day seems a bit daunting, don't worry. In a matter of days it will become second nature. You'll feel as if a new channel has opened in your body that is waiting for you to keep it replenished.

Ideally, start watering your body on a weekend when you are planning to be at home much of the time so that you can easily keep track of how much water you're drinking. Also, because during the first few days you might well find yourself needing to use the loo more often than usual. Don't worry. Your body soon adapts.

Here is all you need:
- An attractive glass which holds 250 ml (8 fl oz).
- A 2-litre (3½-pint) bottle of any natural mineral or spring water you like. Of course, you can drink filtered or unfiltered tap water, but why not treat yourself!

My method is to drink eight of these glasses of water a day, which neatly adds up the 2-litre total you should aim for.

While some people sip water throughout the day, I don't find that it works for me. You also lose count of how much you are drinking and might, optimistically, think you are drinking more than you really are. Eight glasses a day, with each glass holding 250ml (8 fl oz), is easy.

When to drink your 2 litres and why

Naturally, if it's hot, or I have come back from a five-mile walk, I will drink more. The chart below describes a typical day's drinking pattern and it makes sense for three reasons.

1. Drinking two glasses early in the morning helps your body with its process of elimination, so that all the toxins and waste can clear your system.

2. I don't suggest drinking water with meals. That is not to say you shouldn't drink any water with meals; simply that you shouldn't fulfil your daily quota of eight glasses of water by drinking only at meals and nothing at other times during the day. Here's why. If you have a poor appetite and drink at mealtimes, you'll feel bloated from the water and won't be tempted by the food. If you do not have that problem, you will still be concerned about meeting your water quota at meals. Instead of enjoying your food, savouring and chewing every morsel, you will be washing it all down and eating more than you should.

Moreover, water will overload your system if you add it to all the other liquids on offer – soup, wine, followed by coffee, tea and so on. There are a few nutritionists who believe that drinking water with meals dilutes your digestive juices, leading to poor digestion; they too recommend you do not drink water with meals. However, most believe you would need to drink tremendous amounts of water for that to happen. Dr Jane Clarke offers the following advice in 'Taking the Waters' (*The Observer Magazine*, 4 July 1999): 'Water itself does not disturb digestion, but if you fill yourself up with fluid, you'll have less room for food.' She goes on to warn that if you have any digestive disorders, such as a hiatus hernia or inflammation of the oesophagus, 'too much liquid can cause the stomach contents to leak up into the oesophagus [gullet], irritate the oesophagus walls and bring on heartburn.' The way to avoid this is to sip water at mealtimes, not guzzle down glassfuls.

3. The times of day which I have earmarked as best for watering your body coincide with your body's rhythms of high and low energy. Morning is the time to invigorate your body and help it to cleanse itself. Mid-morning, mid-afternoon and early evening are often low-energy times when you need the dynamic, natural element of water to refresh and rejuvenate you. Last thing at night, nothing prepares your body for rest like water, regulating your body temperature and calming you.

**This describes a typical sequence for me, whether on a working day or a holiday.
Try it, or as a close a version of it as you can, until you feel happy drinking the required amount.**

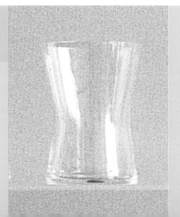

7am

As soon as I open my eyes in the morning I drink my first glass of water, followed in fairly quick succession by my second glass.

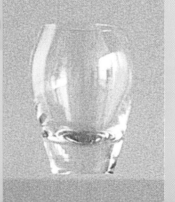

11am

At mid-morning I drink two more glasses of water

3p

Mid-way through the afternoon, I drink two glasses of water.

Drinking water at these times can help you cut down on caffeine and keep you from snacking on quick-fix, high-sugar items which provide very little sustenance. In the brain the receptors for hunger and thirst sit very close together – remember, both are regulated by the hypothalamus. Apparently, signals can easily criss-cross and become confused. This could explain why, when you feel hungry, you minerals in the process. If you put too much caffeine in your system, you will never be able to establish a healthy, stable balance of nutrients, since you will always be excreting them. Many leading nutritionists recommend giving up caffeine and alcohol and, rationally, I am sure they are right. But I love coffee and would find it really hard to give it up. So how could I suggest that you should! As for wine, it has given me up,

You will save yourself hundreds of empty calories each day – if you are drinking natural mineral water, you'll benefit even more.

are actually thirsty: a glass of water, not a bar of chocolate, is what your body needs. Pre-empt your false hunger pangs with a glass of water. You will save yourself hundreds of empty calories each day – if you are drinking natural mineral water, you'll benefit even more.

Coffee, tea and alcohol drain you

If you tend to zero in on wine, coffee or tea whenever you need a lift, you will be less tempted to overindulge if you first slake your thirst with water. Caffeine and alcohol are diuretics which drain your system of vital nutrients. This means that they take more than their own volume of liquid with them as they leave your body, depleting you of important vitamins and

more or less, making me far too susceptible to migraines in exchange for the pleasure of the grape. Make up your own mind. I would simply advise you to limit your cups of coffee or tea to three a day and, if you drink alcohol, give yourself days off on a regular basis.

Be aware, however, that the water you make your tea or coffee with does not count towards your eight glasses (unless it's herbal tea). Only pure water, (with a twist of lemon if you like), will do. Water for chocolate doesn't count either...

See if my method of drinking water at the recommended times works for you. Adjust it to your own schedule until it is comfortable, and do drink all eight glasses. Eat well, get some exercise and lots of sleep. And have a good weekend.

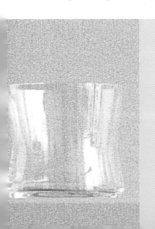

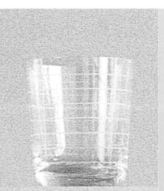

7pm

When I arrive home from work I drink my seventh glass of water.

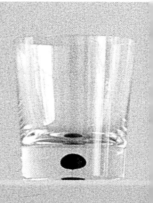

11pm

Just before I go to bed I drink my eighth and last glass of water.

WHICH FOODS HELP TO QUENCH YOUR BODY'S THIRST?

Much as I love potatoes, I have never thought of them as thirst-quenching. In fact 70 per cent of a baked potato is water! So your body can take in quite a bit of water from some of the foods you eat, depending on your diet. If it is a healthy diet and contains plenty of fruits and vegetables, your body will thank you not only for the fibre, vitamins and minerals, but also for the water within them. Look at the table opposite. I've listed some commonly eaten foods (uncooked unless specified) to show you which ones contain a lot, quite a lot, or very little water. Which foods do you eat occasionally, or regularly? You might want to make your own list, noting how much water by percentage each contains. Some, like the potato, are surprising. Others are

to your daily intake. This is because caffeine is a diuretic, causing your body to lose more liquid than the amount you drink. Drinking more than three cups of caffeinated drink a day is not a good idea. Don't blame your water intake for running to the loo – too much caffeine is the culprit!

Alcohol Like caffeine, alcohol is also a diuretic. Each glass of wine you drink needs to be matched with a glass of water to replace lost fluids. A spritzer, a mixture of white wine and sparkling water, usually 50 percent of each, is a good way to do this painlessly, if you like spritzers.

Calories Do you take in more than 2,000 calories daily? Some nutritionists, including Illinois-based Christine Palumbo, RD, advise that you drink one 250ml (8 fl oz) glass

Much as I love potatoes, I have never thought of them as thirst-quenching. In fact 70 per cent of a baked potato is water!

obvious, like watermelon. In each case, calculate how much water your body can expect to draw on during an average three-meals-a-day sequence. Using kitchen scales, weigh your serving of any of the foods listed, then simply multiply the weight, by its percentage of water content. For example, 85g (3oz) of broccoli multiplied by its percentage of water (.90) tells you the amount of water your body gets: 76.5ml (2.7 oz).

Does eating foods with a high water content let you off the hook as far as your daily 2 litres of drinking water are concerned? No – because those two litres are a basic daily minimum, and there are many reasons why you probably need more than that amount. Here are the main ones:

Caffeine For every cup of caffeine-loaded drink (tea, coffee, fizzy – even diet – cola) you will need to add one cup of water

of water for every 250 calories you consume, so 2,000 calories a day means you need eight glasses a day. If you eat more, you should drink more, aiming for nine glasses at the 2,250 level and so on.

Exercise For every 30–45-minute workout, such as swimming or fairly vigorous walking, add one glass to the basic minimum. If you run or play fast sets of tennis, make that two glasses over the basic minimum. Christine Palumbo suggests that if you exercise for an hour or more continuously, you should weigh yourself before and after your workout. For 450g (1lb) of weight lost, add two and a half glasses to your basic minimum.

Pregnancy Check with your doctor, but most advise expectant mothers to take in more than the 2-litre minimum, both by drinking and through the food you eat.

WATER CONTENT OF COMMONLY EATEN FOODS

In general, your diet should top up your daily 2 litres with another 0.5–1 litre (18 fl oz–1¾ pints) of water. Use the table to check whether the foods you eat are quenching your body's need for water. If not, widen your diet to include more water-rich foods. Copy the table and paste it on your fridge to encourage yourself to eat well and embrace the holistic nature of water therapy.

FOOD	PERCENTAGE OF WATER
Romaine lettuce, soya milk, tomatoes, watercress, courgettes	95%
Asparagus, sweet peppers, broccoli, cabbage, cantaloupe melons, carrots, grapefruit, honeydew melons, kale, mushrooms, milk, oranges, orange juice, peaches, spinach, steamed clams, strawberries, unsweetened apple sauce, watermelon	90%
Apples, blueberries, raspberries, kiwi fruit, pears, pineapples, plums, tofu, yogurt	85%
Cherries, cottage cheese, grapes	80%
Avocados, bananas, baked cod, sweetcorn, hard-boiled eggs, ricotta cheese, tuna canned in brine, prawns	75%
Baked potatoes, cooked long-grain rice, white fish (eg. cod, flounder)	70%
Cooked black-eyed beans, roasted skinless chicken, cooked pasta	65%
Chick-peas, ice cream, baked salmon, sirloin steak	60%
Grilled lean beefburgers, reduced-fat mozzarella cheese	50%
White or wholewheat bread, bagels, Cheddar cheese, Swiss cheese	35%
Dry cereal, popped popcorn	less than 5%

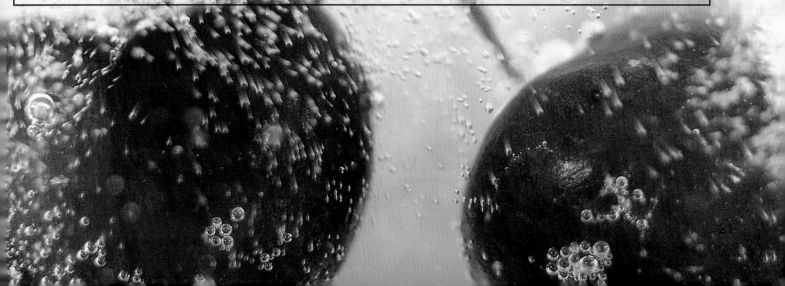

DETOX WITH WATER EVERY DAY AND IN EVERY WAY

This section will help you understand what level of detox you need to undertake and why. I'll show you how water is key to every detox programme, whether it is a carefully worked out, extended version or a daily detox which you are already doing simply by drinking your 2 litres of water .Why is 'doing a detox' suddenly such an 'in' thing? What exactly is it? Do you need to detox? And if so, how often and which kind? It would take several books to answer these questions in full, and some excellent ones which do just that are mentioned in the following pages. Consider, as you read this section, the current state of your own health, what you are willing and able to do to improve it and what you already know and put into practice concerning nutrition and food supplements. All these issues, as well as the latest research into disease prevention and cure, are integrally related to the subject of detoxing your body. It is probably the most important area in health today.

Why is everyone talking about detoxifying?

A tidal wave of concern about environmental pollution, pesticides in food and food allergens, plus the realisation that alcohol, nicotine, medications and drugs, as well as everyday stress, combine literally to *intoxicate* your body on a daily basis, have led to a craze for the opposite – programmes to *detoxify* yourself. These programmes aim to improve your health and deter ageing. If you are 'intoxicating' yourself in one or several ways, the resulting 'unsafe toxins', according to Patrick Holford, 'damage your immune and nervous system, muscles and joints and disrupt hormone balance'. To understand in detail the slippery slope to this unhealthy situation and how to remedy it, read his brilliant book *The Optimum Nutrition Bible.*

What exactly is a 'detox'?

Detoxing aims to cleanse and rid your body of toxins which you take in with food, the air you breathe, or which your own body produces as a result of its digestive and other processes, and which your kidneys then eliminate as waste.

Water is essential to any detox, enabling your body to cleanse itself every day. A detox can be achieved in gradual or dramatic ways: from following a consistent schedule of healthy, balanced meals of unadulterated, organic foods, adding appropriate food supplements, drinking plenty of water and getting exercise and rest, to undergoing a total fast, eating practically nothing and, again, drinking water.

So a detox is a kind of diet (though 'diet' is a commonly misused term denoting weight loss, when it should simply mean a schedule of eating). In any case, you should not detox just to lose weight. You *will* probably lose a few kilos depending on whether or not you are overweight. However, your aim should be to increase health and energy. According to leading nutritionists, detoxing boosts your immune system, thereby preventing illness, and slows down the ageing process.

Holford is 'convinced that toxic overload is often one of the underlying causes of premature senility and maybe Alzheimer's too, as the brain and nervous system cannot detoxify, and start to accumulate toxins'. Preventive medicine is easier and more effective than curing ailments, and he talks about the importance of keeping 'detoxification pathways' clear. If any of the body's ways of eliminating toxins, like your liver, lymphatic system, arteries, veins or kidneys, become overloaded with toxins, your health will suffer. Drinking enough water helps keep these pathways clear. For optimum detox you also need exercise, massage and, as explained in the next section, hydrotherapy: body treatments which can improve circulation.

Both your lymphatic and veinous systems (your veins as opposed to arteries) are fairly static and need stimulation to keep the fluids flowing through them. This is why it is a good idea to perform 'body brushing', (see page 64) every day. Lymphatic massage, done professionally at spas, is also beneficial. (In contrast to the static lymphatic and veinous systems, arterial blood is pumped around your body by your heart, and although your arteries can become blocked, the arterial system is nonetheless 'motored' by your heart.)

Reduced cellulite, weight loss, a clearer complexion and lowered stress levels will gradually be achieved if you stay with your daily detox – depending on your current state of health and how determined you are.

Do not do a detox thinking it is a crash diet. You shouldn't crash diet anyway – not only is it unhealthy, it doesn't work. (Read Marilyn Glenville's motivating and sensible book *Natural Alternatives to Dieting*.) Try to understand what your body needs and then follow it through. If I have learned one thing in my research for this book, it is that to achieve results in the area of health, beauty and fitness, you have to take a holistic approach. Whether you are watering your body internally or externally, it is essential to integrate those methods with good nutrition and exercise, and to find effective ways of relaxing.

So you need to detox daily – but do you also need to detox more intensely?

You certainly need to keep your system detoxified for all the reasons above. Follow a basic day-to-day regime of a healthy, balanced diet (preferably organic), limit your caffeinated drinks to three cups a day and drink a minimum of 2 litres of water daily, fulfilling the rest of your body's water needs with

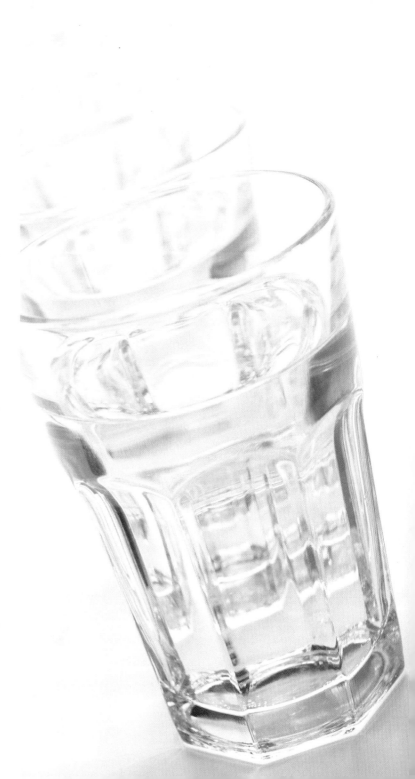

water-rich foods. (Alcohol is never part of any detox, so if you choose to include it in your day-to-day life, make sure you always top up with water, glass for glass. Limit your intake in any case, give your body 'days off' so that it can cleanse itself – and don't overload it with other polluting and toxic factors.)

There are various detoxes you can intersperse with your basic day-to-day one. Some are fairly easy to follow over a weekend, others last ten days, a month, or just one day. At the extreme end of the scale there is the total fast, which has religious overtones of purification stemming from Jesus's forty-day fast in the desert. Which – if any – should you do?

The total fast

Easily the most controversial is the total fast. Most nutritionists believe that it is too drastic for your body to go without food for days. According to John Garrow, a retired professor of nutrition: 'Fasting is potentially dangerous, because it is so easily abused. It offers rigid control over food intake, which is what anorexics find attractive.' Dr Susan Jebb from the Medical Research Council's Dunn Nutrition Laboratory in Cambridge points out how unsuccessful these supervised fasts were in treating obese people – their lost weight was soon put on again. But weight loss is not the point of a fast – just as any detox should not be done just to lose weight. Dr Ian Drysdale, principal of the British College of Naturopathy and Osteopathy, sees fasting as a valuable means of giving the body a rest. However, he too concludes that overall he is against a long fast for two very important reasons:

● The build-up of pollutants harmlessly stored in the body's fatty tissue – a method your body apparently cleverly figured out to keep those toxins away from your vital organs – can be suddenly released into your bloodstream on a crash diet or prolonged fast.

● Most people don't have time to carry out a long fast safely.

The mono-fast

What about the less drastic detoxes? Many regimes begin with, or contain within a week-long or month-long detox, what is called a 'mono-fast' or fruit fast, but you could try this on its own. It involves eating a single fruit all day – hence mono – along with drinking at least 2 litres of water. You can eat as much of the chosen (preferably organic) fruit as you like, in four or five 'meals'. It can be rather boring, though you can switch fruits at mid-day if you wish, but the theory is that one fruit all day gives your digestive system less to 'think about' and allows it to rest – an important principle of all detox programmes. So if you are going to do it, you might as well do it right! Each fruit offers different concentrations of vitamins and minerals. The pectin in apples, for example, is excellent for detoxification and, according to Leslie Kenton, 'also helps prevent protein matter in the intestines from putrefying'. You may want to do a one-day mono-fast trying each fruit individually, say twice a month over the year. Some people do this detox once a week – it certainly is easy and good for you.

You may nonetheless be determined to go ahead with a prolonged detox. What should you expect? Most people doubtless begin with every good intention. The first day goes well. It's tough, but hey! – it's a detox, not a party: it's meant to be tough. On the second day, when the crashing headache refuses to go, most people head for two paracetamol and a glass of water. By evening, clear-headed at last and slightly dizzy, when they feel food beginning to beckon, the weak-willed succumb to a fridge raid. Following a strict detox diet is not easy, especially if you are working hard. It is much easier to undergo a long regime at a spa where you are being cared for and catered to, where you can rest and relax. Starting programmes and not finishing them is always demotivating, making you less likely to try simple methods which you can achieve.

However, if you would like to try a prolonged detox, you could follow Jane Scrivner's rigorous thirty-day plan which she outlines in her book *Detox Yourself*. She promises that you can lose weight, boost your immune system, reduce your cellulite, look younger and be so full of energy that your life will be extended by an hour a day. Scrivner co-founded the British School of Complementary Therapy, so her approach is holistic. She recommends thirty minutes of exercise, skin brushing and drinking 2 litres of water a day – things you should do every day anyway.

A shorter, very sensible programme is Leslie Kenton's '10 Day Spring Clean' which she details in *10 Steps to a New You*. It is based largely on a raw-food diet and will launch you into healthy eating habits if you need a bit of encouragement.

Water: the common factor

All detox programmes share one element: water. You can live without food for days, but not without water. Only water has the ability to flush out waste and toxins, not only from your kidneys, but also from every pore of your skin and with every exhalation of breath. If you are drinking 2 litres of water every day, you are already flushing out toxins. Perhaps all you need is an adjustment – minor or major – to your daily diet and exercise routine to accomplish gradually but permanently improved levels of health and fitness.

Maintaining a healthy regime

Whatever detox plan you choose, do not return to an intoxicating diet. Cut down on caffeine and alcohol and on saturated fats (particularly in meat and dairy products), cut out refined sugar and all refined carbohydrates, eat plenty of fruit and vegetables (steamed or raw) and drink lots of water. Exercise at least three times a week and get enough sleep. A sensible diet, plenty of water, exercise, sleep: it is the ancient and modern mantra of good health. Water is pure therapy, enabling your body to eliminate waste and toxins, carrying nutrients to every cell and feeding you with its own minerals.

As well as playing a vital role in detoxifying, water also replenishes you – especially mineral water, as you'll see in the following section. So as you go through the course of a day drinking your 2 litres, you will be replenishing as well as detoxifying your system, hour by hour, gently and naturally. I think of this internal watering of the body as a parallel to the ocean's ebb and flow: day after day, the tide shifts acres of sand and pebbles, clearing the beach of debris, while cleansing itself from within with purifying seaweed. Ah, but not all beaches are clean, you say! And you are right. This is because not even the ocean can always cope with all of debris thrown into it. And neither can your body.

A bit of junk food won't kill you! However, if you smoke, drink lots of alcohol and caffeine, make do with pre-prepared food, prefer refined carbohydrates to wholegrain bread and pasta, skimp on fruit and vegetables, eat nothing organic, take little or no exercise, get insufficient sleep and drink no water, you will be subjecting your body to toxins and pesticides which it cannot easily eliminate, as well as robbing it of nutrients.

Do this every day, year in year out and you will need more than a detox or a glass of water to set you on the right track.

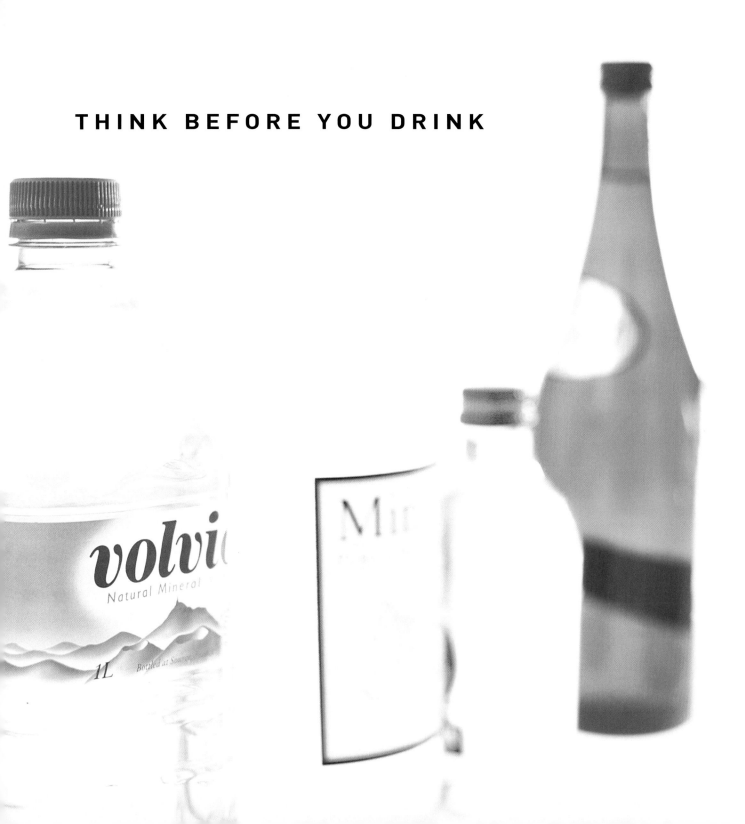

THINK BEFORE YOU DRINK

'I'll show thee the best springs;

I'll pluck thee berries;

I'll fish for thee and get thee wood enough' "

THE TEMPEST
WILLIAM SHAKESPEARE

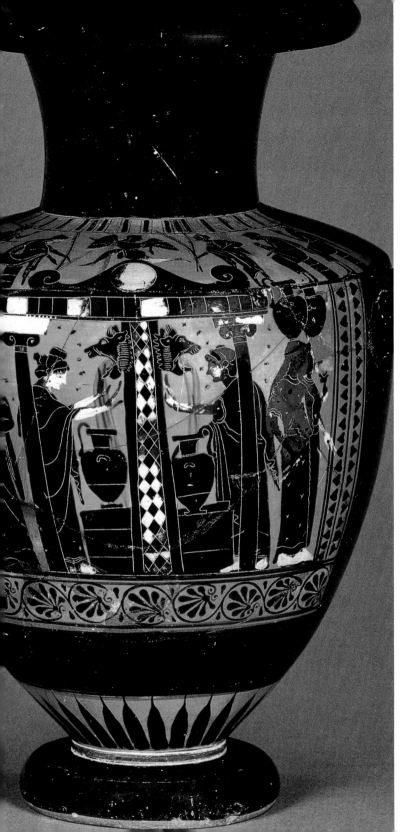

If you were wandering the earth thousands of years ago looking for an ideal place to settle, your final decision, like that of our earliest ancestors, would be largely determined by access to fresh, uncontaminated water. A fast-flowing stream or river, a sparkling lake – any of these would attract you.

They would guarantee plentiful water for you and your animals to drink. In desert or dry areas where rain was unreliable, you would depend on a nearby water source for bathing, cooking, cleaning, and for growing your crops. Water would offer you protein-rich fish and shellfish.

What if you found a spring, where water came bubbling miraculously out of the ground! That would be truly precious – even sacred. A spring is an unfailing source of clean, fresh water and less likely than a river or lake to be contaminated by human or animal activity. And if that spring were in a wood near the sea?

'I'll show thee the best springs; I'll pluck thee berries; I'll fish for thee and get thee wood enough.'

In giving Caliban these lines in *The Tempest*, Shakespeare was describing a rural idyll which no longer exists: an ideal site for people to live and, moreover, to flourish.

It is no surprise that Knossos, the largest of the great Minoan palaces, was built in a fertile valley on Crete's north coast, with wood for building, the sea for communication and a continuous supply of uncontaminated spring water for drinking. This labyrinthine palace complex was for nearly two thousand years the key political, economic, artistic and religious centre of the Minoan civilisation, lasting from around 3000 to 1375 BC.

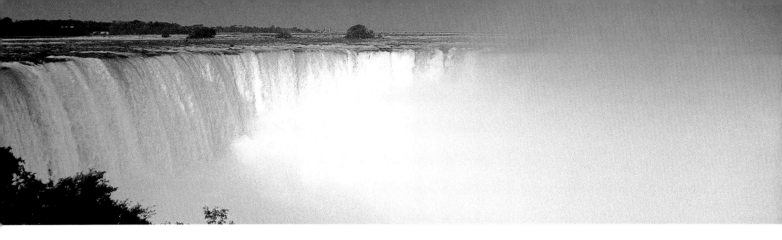

The earliest towns and cities also sprang up near ready sources of fresh water. The ancient cities of Babylon and Ur on the River Euphrates, Byblos on the sea in Lebanon, thought to be the world's oldest continuously occupied city, as well as ancient cities on the North Indian plain and in China, were all close to fresh water supplies. Biblical Jerusalem was founded on the Gihon Spring, though by the eighth century BC King Hezekiah of Israel had built underground aqueducts to bring water to his growing capital from sources many kilometres away. Only a century or two later, in the mountains of Persia (now Iran), a system of gently down-sloping tunnels drilled into groundwater deposits, known as *qanats*, extracted water for the thickly populated plains. The water was distributed by gravity along a network of brick channels. Until 1933 Teheran, Iran's capital, still relied on these pre-Christian *qanats*. Ancient Rome's water supply, with its hundreds of miles of enclosed aqueducts and huge reservoirs, was one of the wonders of the world.

Whenever large numbers of human beings lived together in settlements, the big question became – and still is – not so much where to get fresh water but to do with the waste?

In a city, two vital tasks must be undertaken: drinking water must be brought to us and our waste taken away. The two must never be allowed to mingle or sickness will result.

Our ancestors had no germ theory of disease, though common sense told them to develop methods to deal with obviously foul water. In fact, there are Sanskrit records dating back to 2000 BC showing how to purify water through boiling and filtering. Ancient Rome was frequently wracked by cholera and typhus epidemics. Outbreaks of waterborne disease spread to this day with terrifying swiftness in parts of Africa, in refugee camps and in any chronically, or suddenly overcrowded, area. Until the 1850s, waterborne epidemics made cities like London unhealthy places.

In the nineteenth century, as the urban populations in Europe and America exploded, science brought two crucial advances. Cholera, lethal scourge of the cities, was defeated by the building of modern sewers which carefully separated drinking water and waste. Meanwhile the German scientist Robert Koch finally identified the tiny organisms – germs – which led to infection.

Within only two or three generations, improvements in drainage, water treatment and sanitation had transformed people's lives. Death rates in Western countries plummeted and average life expectancy doubled. Civilisation flourished.

Now you can trust the water that flows from your tap to be safe, but you may want to drink it from other sources, and not just because it's fashionable.

HOW HEALTHY IS THE WATER YOU ARE DRINKING?

This is a book about how to feel and look your best – how to use the pure therapy of water to help you achieve and maintain optimum levels of health and well-being all day and every day. So this section on drinking water is not about what is and isn't safe: your water company can report on that.

You want to know which waters will do you positive good. Water itself will indeed benefit you – 'quantity rather than quality is the key to success', according to Dr Jane Clarke. And despite the concerns I will be sharing with you about what is in tap water, I certainly agree that drinking tap water is better than drinking no water at all.

mineral water for all cooking purposes, so I suggest using jug-filtered water for making coffee, tea and ice cubes, and for all cooking. I recommend drinking only natural mineral water. It is expensive, I resent that I cannot drink delicious, health-giving water straight from my tap. Nonetheless I am lucky to live in a country where tap water is safe and plentiful. That's the current situation, so I make my choices accordingly.

Read the following pages carefully. Consider your needs. You'll find a dos and don'ts list at the end of this section, as well as two tables detailing the mineral contents of the various bottled waters available in the shops – all to help you enjoy your daily 2 litres.

It would be impossibly expensive to use natural mineral water for all cooking purposes, so I suggest using jug-filtered water for making coffee, tea and ice cubes, and for all cooking.
I recommend drinking only natural mineral water.

This is true for the same reasons that nutritionists advise you to eat plenty of fresh fruit and vegetables, even though much of the produce you find on supermarket shelves has been sprayed with pesticides and fungicides whose long-term effect on the human body is unknown. Quite simply, the benefits outweigh the risks.

However, just as it makes sense to buy organic or traditionally grown produce if you can find (and afford) it, it is worth drinking the best, least processed water you can get, water which offers you the best balance of minerals you need. It would be impossibly expensive to use natural

How your water is made safe for drinking.

We in the so-called developed countries of the world have largely banished 'natural' dangers from our water, though in less technologically advanced countries unsafe water is still a critical problem with potentially tragic consequences. According to Oxfam, millions die throughout Asia and Africa, especially children, from common diseases often spread by the consumption of contaminated water. In Sudan, for example, £2 a month would help provide enough tools for villagers to dig a well and give them a permanent supply of clean, safe water.

In developed countries the chief concerns are chemical contamination – from industrial processes (including modern farming), as well as from the chemicals used to 'clean' our water, ironically enough.

It is, perhaps, unreasonable to expect that the water you use – at a rate of 73 litres (16 gallons) a day on average – for all domestic purposes should also be perfect, by which I mean beneficial as well as safe for drinking. To produce the required quantities to that level would be fabulously expensive, even technically impossible. Let's start with safe.

The mains water that comes out of your tap usually goes through four basic processes before it is considered safe for domestic consumption:

grained, dense mineral, garnet. There are also pressure-filters which involve water being pumped through a cylindrical steel tank, though these are more common for industrial use and for large public swimming pools.

● Disinfection, the most important (to protect you from waterborne diseases) but also most the problematic. The cheapest, most widely used method involves chlorine (also found in household bleaches and disinfectants). But chlorines can combine with other naturally occurring substances to produce chloroform and other harmful compounds. Other processes use ozone gases (safer but complicated to produce and more expensive) or ultraviolet radiation which is completely without side effects but very expensive.

It is perhaps unreasonable to expect that the water you use – at a rate of 73 litres (16 gallons) a day on average – for all domestic purposes should also be perfect, by which I mean beneficial as well as safe for drinking.

● Sedimentation, where it rests in huge tanks until most impurities have sunk to the bottom and can be disposed of.
● Coagulation and flocculation, in which lighter, undissolved impurities are treated with chemicals which cause them to stick to each other in larger, heavier masses of solids called 'floc'. These are then subjected to further mixing before being pushed into the sedimentation tanks to settle with the other solids.
● Filtration, which catches any remaining solids (which can shield microbes from disinfection). Most modern filters work on layers of anthracite coal, fine sand and often of the fine-

The good news is that your mains water is 'safe' in that it carries no disease or other immediate threats to your health. The so-so news? The water from your tap probably tastes flat, it may have been robbed of beneficial minerals and could well smell like the local swimming pool. The bad news is that there is increasing reason to believe that some of the very chemicals used to make your water 'safe' may cause long-term harm. You can filter tap water in a variety of ways to make it better (see pages 34–5). However, when it comes to drinking your daily 2 litres, you just might want to become a bottled water baby.

THE INS AND OUTS OF TAP WATER

What is in your tap water?

Studies in America and Canada have led to suspicions that trihalomethanes in drinking water (some of the chloroform by-products of chlorination) may increase the chances of foetal abnormalities and of cancers of the bladder, colon and rectum. According to the *Toronto Star*, a conference in 1996 was told that up to 500 cases of cancer and 140 deaths in Ontario alone could be attributable to chlorine in drinking water. Water authorities in the USA, Europe and Britain have all recently set lower limits for these compounds (100 parts per billion) – but, given their extremely toxic nature, is the

commercial petrol. It did indeed help 'clean, lean' burning of fuel in our car engines. The trouble was, evidence soon began to accumulate that this relatively untested chemical's volatile nature, its small molecular size and its solubility in water were causing it to get to places where gasoline alone could not go. Motor boats were spreading it into lakes and rivers; fuel tank and pipe leaks were allowing it to seep into underground wells, aquifers and water supplies.

At first the oil companies and the US government's Environmental Protection Agency claimed that the chemical was not dangerous. By 1998, however, it was obvious that thousands of wells, lakes and other sources of drinking water

Since you'll be drinking 2 litres of water a day, unfiltered tap water isn't your healthiest option.

only really safe level zero?

Another additive to tap water that is causing concern is aluminium sulphate which is used to remove impurities such as clay particles from tap water. A government-funded study in south-western France found that increased residues of aluminium sulphate correlated almost exactly with rates of increase for Alzheimer's Disease in the local population. Meanwhile, at the UK's Sussex University a scientist believes that one in ten children suffer from learning and behavioural difficulties as a result of exposure to lead in the environment, and that the main sources are old lead-based paints and the lead pipes still used to carry mains water to large areas of the UK.

Even the well-meaning health lobby has helped to create new dangers. In the early 1990s, after a long campaign by environmentalists, leaded petrol began to be banned or phased out. As a result, MTBE (methyl tertiary-butyl ether), a by-product of the oil-refining process, began to be added to

were becoming poisoned. Worrying press reports began to appear. The *San Francisco Chronicle* described MTBE leaks as 'a ticking time-bomb' and a threat to the nation's water supply.

Early in 1999 a thorough investigation by the American group Communities for a Better Environment turned the tide. In March of that year the Governor of California banned the use of MTBE in petrol; Connecticut and several other states rapidly followed suit. And by the way, after first denying it, a British oil company confessed that it is indeed building a plant for producing MTBE in the UK.

Finally, there are still pesticide residues in much of our tap water. In the UK about a quarter of all mains water contains these in excess of European Union maximum admissible concentrations.

So what is emerging from your tap is not ideal. Since you'll be drinking 2 litres of water a day, unfiltered tap water may not be your healthiest option.

What is not in your tap water?

This is also an important question, because water can do more than just irrigate and cleanse your body. It is in many ways your body's most important nutrient and, like any healthy food, can actively replenish your body's store of minerals. You are much more likely to be deficient in minerals than say, protein, and water is an easy way to boost your levels of the major and the trace minerals.

Calcium Water has been shown to be as effective as milk in transmitting the benefits of calcium, so why drink from a supply where this vital element is either not present or has been all but eradicated? For example, if you live in a soft-

understandable reasons) see water provision as primarily a safety issue rather than a positive health opportunity.

Don't drink distilled water

It sounds tempting, doesn't it – water absolutely purified and with all solids and toxins taken out? That's the trouble with it. 'Pure' is not necessarily healthy. Distilled water not only tastes terrible, it lacks all the health-enhancing minerals you need. And, to make matters worse, because pure water looks to bond with other substances on its trip through your body (to complete its own molecular structure), it leaches the minerals from your body, actually stealing the minerals your

Water has been shown to be as effective as milk in transmitting the benefits of calcium.

water area where the water is low on natural minerals, and you are drinking your 2 litres a day, your tap water may be supplying you with as little as 30 mg of calcium per day. Your body's minimum daily requirement is 600 mg. Yet the equivalent amount of the average natural spring water (by American classification) contains in excess of 100 mg of bone-building calcium, giving you more than three times as much. Water can be a calorie-free source of calcium every day!

Magnesium This mineral is essential to keep your heart and circulation healthy, as well as helping to maintain strong bones and teeth. You will not come across magnesium in much tap water. In fact, it may have been removed. Recent research in the USA has led to alarm over magnesium deficiencies in the general diet and even to demands that magnesium be added to water in much the same way as fluoride. However, the water companies (for perfectly

body already contains.

Distilled water is an important temporary resource in dealing with specific medical conditions (and is excellent for keeping irons unclogged), but the consensus is quite simple and damning: as part of your daily requirement, distilled water could do more harm than good.

Don't be a softie

The same goes for water softeners: the results are lovely for rinsing your hair or making the family's clothes wash fluffier, but worse than useless for drinking. Most commercial softeners remove beneficial minerals and replace them with sodium – at a time when you are probably trying to cut down on the amount of sodium in your diet!

All of which leads to the next question: what can you do to make your tap water healthier if you choose to drink what's on tap for your daily 2 litres?

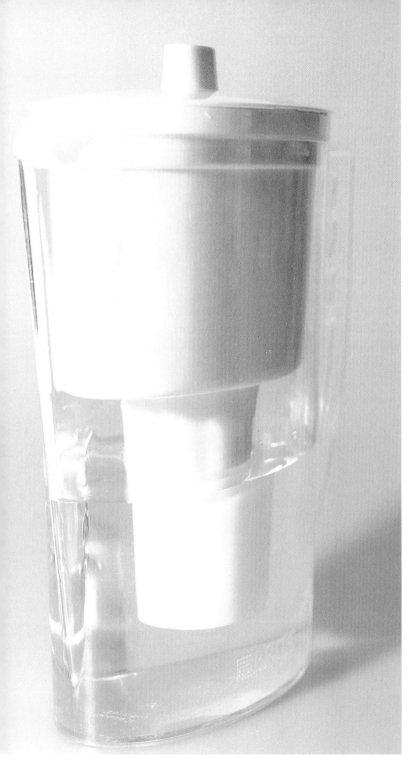

TAP INTO THE BEST FILTERS

If you cannot get your water from a guaranteed untainted source, be sure you filter it before drinking it or cooking with it, to minimise problems with solids, nitrates, chlorine, pesticides and other common pollutants that may have evaded the treatment process. Here is a summary of the home water-filtering devices that are easy to use, some more affordable than others.

Jug filter

The simple, portable operation that you fill from the tap. It requires a replaceable carbon filter cartridge (£2–3 each).* This is what I use at the moment for filtering tap water for cooking, for making tea and coffee and also for ice cubes – why add frozen tap water to your glass of expensive mineral water? I've invested in a toughened glass jug (between £20 and £30) because I don't like the way plastic discolours, but plastic jugs (about £10) are fine for the purpose. Keep the jug in the fridge and use the water within twenty-four hours of filtration.

Advantages? The jugs are cheap (though the cost of the filter cartridges can mount up). Carbon filters leave in many of the healthy minerals you need, yet screen out chlorine and other unwelcome chemicals, enhancing tap water's clarity and taste.

Drawbacks? Carbon filters do not block out bacteria or microbes. And they have to be changed quite frequently, usually after you have filtered between 50 and 200 litres (10 and 44 gallons) of water, depending on the type of cartridge. It is most important to change the cartridges according to the manufacturer's instructions as they lose their permeability and can become a breeding-place for germs.

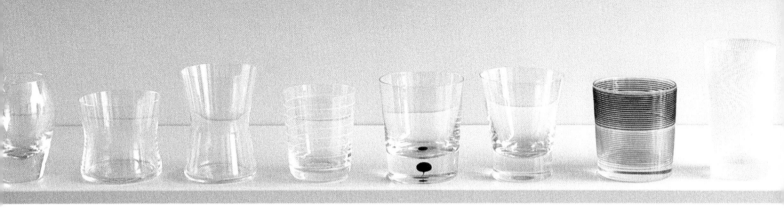

'Point of use' system

This device is installed next to the kitchen sink, either on or below a work surface. Most supply a separate tap from which you take your drinking water. They use activated carbon filters and are obviously suitable if you want to treat larger quantities of water. They cost between £50 and £200 to buy, £20 to £50 to install and £20 to £80 annually for cartridges.*Also available in this category are systems which feature combined ceramic and activated carbon filters. The ceramic filters consist of very fine clay particles which have the added advantage of removing some harmful micro-organisms and particles. They cost about the same to buy and run as the carbon-only devices. Again, these systems enhance water quality without screening out most of the healthful salts and minerals.

Reverse osmosis system

This system was originally invented in order to desalinate sea water and cleanse it of impurities. The units now sold for domestic use can also be fitted near your sink, as with 'point of use' systems, though they may require the installation of an extra storage tank to collect the treated water. The system works by forcing some of the water through a semi-permeable membrane, which allows small molecules such as water to pass through but flushes away the contaminants with the rest of the water.

Reverse osmosis is probably the most efficient system in terms of removing potentially health-endangering substance impurities, chemicals and bacteria. Unfortunately it also removes the salts and minerals that your body needs. Moreover, it discards four fifths of the water, is very slow and normally needs a particle pre-filter to be fitted as well. This is also the most expensive of the kitchen-use systems, costing £300–700 to buy, £50–70 to plumb in and £60–140 a year to run. If your water pressure is less than ideal, you may need a pump too. For most people, this system probably amounts to overkill.

Speaking of which, if you are especially worried about nitrates (agricultural fertiliser residues) in your drinking water, you can also buy units which remove these and replace them with chlorides (£50–200 to buy, £100 to install with cartridges at £30–50 apiece).

Like many water softeners, these may also use salt and add sodium to your water, which can raise blood pressure and cause water retention in the body.

*All figures from *Which?* magazine, January 1998.

LEARN THE LANGUAGE OF BOTTLED WATERS

There is a very well put-together, informative website on the Internet entitled www.bottledwaterweb.com. It deals, as its name implies, with the world of bottled waters, principally in the USA but also globally. Of course, since it is supported by bottled water manufacturers, you would want to cross-check the website's information with other sources. The IBWA (International Bottled Water Association) site, at www.bottledwater.org is also very useful. For specifically European information, refer to www.naturalmineralwater.org. But the more you investigate, the more people you talk to, the more you look at what the lyrical descriptions actually mean, the more it becomes clear (with apologies to the excellent websites) that the international bottled water marketplace is indeed a tangled web. I'll help you untangle it.

You may have become so distrustful of your mains water supply that you are tempted by the first pretty bottle on your supermarket's shelf, with its visions of green hills, snowy mountains or pellucid raindrops, and accept that the water behind the label must be special, healthy or 'pure', particularly when the blurb describes it as 'spring water', 'mineral water', 'table water' or even 'mountain dew'. After all, how could it be worse than tap water?

Big mistake. It is not that manufacturers lie. It's simply that you do have to learn the language of bottled waters to see clearly beyond the label.

It is perfectly legal to sink a well into groundwater, exploit a spring or lake or river, even to buy water from municipal or commercial sources and put it in bottles. Then – as long as the water reaches certain minimum treatment standards – you can sell it at a price vastly exceeding that of its production. The resulting product may be inferior in taste and quality to your local tap water. It may contain fewer minerals and other beneficial elements. So don't buy anything until you have read these pages. You'll understand what all the labels mean and you will be able to distinguish what the water you are paying extra for offers you. It's easy once you know how.

In the USA and most of Europe (including the UK), certain descriptions applied to bottled water are strictly controlled. Look for the precise words on the label of the bottled water, according to where you live, to ensure that you are getting the water you're paying for.

- In Europe the key phrase is: 'natural mineral water'.
- In the USA and Canada there are two key phrases: 'natural spring water' and 'natural mineral water'.

What do these phrases mean? The law in the EU, now fully extended to the UK, describes natural mineral water as:

'...microbiologically wholesome water originating in an underground water table or deposit and emerging from a spring tapped at one or more natural or bore exits. Natural mineral water can be distinguished from ordinary drinking water, notably:

a) by its nature, which is characterised by its mineral content, trace elements and other constituents.

b) by its original state.'

Before being bottled and sold, any natural mineral water must be subjected to two years of analysis to ensure that its mineral content remains constant, and details of the source and contents must also be made available (most reputable companies print these on the bottle label). Further, the waters must be 'protected from all risk of pollution in order to preserve intact these characteristics'.

A 1996 amendment to the EU regulations tightened up

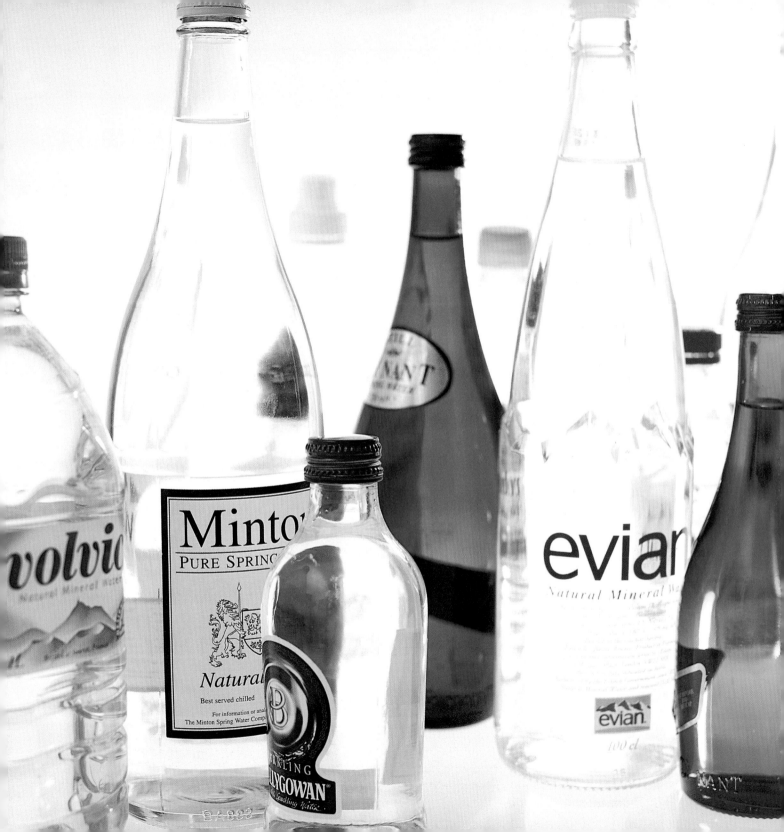

mineral water definitions and also laid down conditions for what can be called 'spring water'. The key change from recent legislation is that spring waters must now also be microbiologically stable. It must also be bottled at source. In the UK this has resulted in relabelling of some of the more dubious 'spring water' products. However, spring water, unlike natural mineral water, can still be subject to certain treatments, including the removal of certain minerals to make the water safe to drink. Natural mineral water must emerge from the ground already safe to drink with consistent and safe levels of minerals. Natural mineral water therefore remains the only water in Europe that is guaranteed to be naturally pure and wholesome, without *any* treatment, except for the addition of carbon dioxide in some cases.

Benjamin Franklin (wearing his entrepreneurial hat) was the first to import mineral water into the USA over two hundred years ago.

The boom in the last twenty years has seen local and imported 'mineral waters' on the market, but they are still overwhelmed by various other local forms of bottled water, which may or may not be from 'pure' sources. The US Food and Drug Administration oversees the production of water sold in bottles or other containers (which are categorised as a 'food'), while the Environmental Protection Agency is responsible for regulating tap water (legally defined as a 'utility'). The FDA is generally recognised as the toughest, most thorough regulator in the food world, so it is worth running through how it categorises the various waters. The

Don't pay extra for bottles labelled 'table water'. They can come from just about anywhere, though they must meet certain hygienic standards.

Don't pay extra for bottles labelled 'table water'. They can come from just about anywhere, though they must meet certain hygienic standards. On balance, table water is probably not preferable to tap water, especially if the latter is properly filtered.

Regulating bottled water in the USA

In the USA, the situation is more complex. America has a long tradition of bottled waters – early travellers and settlers needed guaranteed sources of safer water – but until recently they were more of a convenience than a health drink. Only the elite drank European-style 'mineral waters' for their health. In fact, eighteenth-century American statesman and polymath

following is a brief summary of the descriptions that must appear on the bottles (for a fuller version see the IBWA website at www.bottledwater.org):

Artesian water\artesian well water Bottled water from a well that taps a confined aquifer (a water-bearing underground layer of rock or sand) in which the water level stands at some height above the top of the aquifer.

Drinking water Another name for bottled water – that is, water that is sold for human consumption in sanitary containers and contains no added sweeteners or chemical additives (other than flavours, extracts or essences – not to comprise more than 1 per cent by weight of the final product, which will otherwise be called a soft drink).

Mineral water Bottled water containing not less than 250 parts per million total dissolved solids may be labelled as mineral water. It is distinguished from other bottled waters by its constant level and relative proportions of mineral and trace elements at the point of emergence from the source. No minerals can be added.

Purified water Water that has been produced by distillation, deionisation, reverse osmosis or other suitable processes and that meets the definition of purified water in the United States Pharmacopoeia. Other suitable product names for bottled water treated by one of the above processes include 'distilled water' if produced by distillation, 'deionised water' if the process used is deionisation, or 'reverse osmosis water' if the process is reverse osmosis.

Confusingly for Europeans, in the USA 'spring water' can mean 'mineral water'. There the classification of 'natural mineral water' is especially tough and excludes many low-mineral European brands which weigh in at less than the 250 parts per million (the same as mg per litre) mentioned above. So you could find your favourite natural mineral water in a European country labelled as a natural spring water in the USA.

For example, Evian – marketed in the EU and elsewhere in the world as a 'natural mineral water' – reaches 309 parts per million. For waters between 250 and 500 parts per million, the FDA gives producers an alternative: to describe their product as 'natural mineral water' or 'natural spring water'. The Evian USA spokesman I consulted at the time of

...you could find your favourite natural mineral water in a European country labelled as a natural spring water in the US.

Sparkling water Water that after treatment and possible replacement with carbon dioxide contains the same amount of carbon dioxide that it had at emergence from the source. (Soda water, seltzer water and tonic water are not considered bottled waters. They are regulated separately, may contain sugar and calories, and are considered soft drinks.)

Spring water Bottled water derived from an underground formation from which water flows naturally to the surface of the earth. Spring water must be collected only at the spring or through a bore hole tapping the underground formation.

Well water Bottled water from a hole bored, drilled or otherwise constructed in the ground which taps the water of an aquifer.

writing this book said that the company chooses to label Evian as 'natural spring water' in America because, particularly outside the major cities, 'mineral water' is generally associated with a sparkling rather than a still drink. However, in America any bottled water containing in excess of 500 parts per million dissolved solids *must* describe itself as 'natural mineral water'.

For my daily 2 litres in the UK, I simply look for 'natural mineral water'. If I'm in the USA I either stay with a brand I know and trust, or, if I'm experimenting with new brands, I read the label to check that it is low in both sodium and nitrates. Look at the tables on page 40–1 to choose the water for you.

THERE IS MINERAL WEALTH IN YOUR WATER

There is long tradition of travelling to British and European spas and 'taking the waters' at source for their promised medicinal benefits. Now there is a high-tech industry that brings the spas' waters to us. The bottled mineral-water boom hit London in the early 1980s when, suddenly, parties were awash not only with wine, but water. And, interestingly these bottled waters are leading many of us back to the spas.

France has had strict rules in place with regard to mineral water for over a hundred years, perhaps because it has always been part of the culture, and it is also a major export. My personal preference is for French mineral waters, but waters from Italy, Germany, Sweden, Ireland, North America and, of course, the UK are also carefully regulated. How should you choose one? Flavour and provenance. Simply decide what mineral content you want or need and then taste various brands. (These are not choices you have with the water from your tap.) In America and Britain, drinking waters for their mineral content is fairly new. So you may want to start with a low-mineral brand and then move on to the more continental approach with a high mineral content, because you would like to replace or supplement your morning round of shiny little pills. In all these cases there is a mineral water for you.

Here are two tables, the first showing the exact mineral composition of a selection of well-known brands (domestic and imported) in the UK and the second grading them in an at-a-glance way according to their overall mineral content.

MINERAL COMPOSITION OF NATURAL MINERAL WATERS (MG/LITRE)

brand	Sodium	Calcium	Magnesium	Potassium	Nitrates	Chloride	Sulphates	Fluoride	Silica	Bicarbonate
Abbey Well	45	54	35	7.5	0.9	80	28	0.09	–	173
Apollinaris	556.1	47.5	124	321.2	187.7	–	142.1	0.35	21.6	1962.0
Aqua-Pura	22	35	5.3	2.2	34	38	22	0.1	–	–
Ashbourne	10	102	241	3	0.4	30	60	0.2	8.6	329.0
Badoit	150	190	85	10	18.0	40	40	1.3	30.0	1100.0
Ballygowan	15.4	121.2	18.6	2.8	9.2	24.8	22.6	0.1	7.0	451.4
Brecon Carreg	5.7	47.5	16.5	0.4	2.2	13	9	0.1	6.0	90.0
Bru	10	23.3	22.6	1.8	0.5	4.0	3.5	0.1	15.0	209.0
Buxton	24	55	19	1	0.1	42	23	–	–	248
Chiltern Hills	9	101	2.1	1	6.4	14	4.9	0.1	–	299
Contrexeville	9.1	486	84	3.2	1	8.6	1187	0.3	8.1	386.0
Cwm Dale	7.1	13.1	3	0.5	12	7.9	10.4	0.12	8.2	37.0
Evian	5	78	24	1	3.8	4.5	10	0.12	13.5	357.0
Ferrarelle	41	448.2	21.3	39	4.5	23.5	3.6	0.7	97.8	1586.0
Highland Spring	6	35	8.5	0.6	1	7.5	6	0.1	9.3	180.6
Malvern	14	37	19	1.5	7.1	43.5	24.5	0.15	8.5	127.0
Naya	6	38	22	–	0.5	1	17	–	–	243.0
Perrier	9	147.3	3.4	1	18.3	21.5	33	0.1	12.0	347.7
Poland Spring	2.9	8.3	0.8	0.5	–	6.1	5	–	–	20.0
Ramlosa	190	1.8	0.5	1.7	0.3	28	1213	3.5	7.7	556.0
San Pellegrino	45	207	58	2.3	0.6	–	540	0.56	10.5	231.0
Spa Barisart	5	5.5	1.5	0.5	1.5	5.5	7.5	0.1	10.0	18.0
Spa Reine	3	3.5	1.3	0.5	1.9	5	6.5	0.1	7.0	11.0
Vichy Celestins	1292	109	11.7	71.5	1.2	230	136	5.6	36.0	3367.0
Vichy St Yorre	1132	34	7.5	88	1	202	102	3.0	1415.0	2915.0
Vittel Bonne	7.3	91	19.9	4.9	0.6	–	105	–	–	258.0
Volvic	9.4	9.9	6.1	5.7	6.3	8.4	6.9	0.3	30.0	64.0

Source: manufacturers' analyses

MINERAL WATERS ARRANGED IN ORDER OF MINERAL CONTENT

Highest mineral content	Medium mineral content
Vichy Celestins (France)	Malvern (UK)
Vichy St Yorre (France)	Abbey Well (UK)
Apollinaris (Germany)	Bru (UK)
Contrexeville (France)	Vittel Bonne Source (France)
Ramlösa (Sweden)	Buxton (UK)
Ferrarelle (Italy)	Chiltern Hills (UK)
San Pellegrino (Italy)	Brecon (UK)
Badoit (France)	Volvic (France)
Ashbourne (UK)	Aqua-Pura (UK)
Perrier (France)	Spa Reine (Belgium)
Ballygowan (Ireland)	Spa Barisart (Belgium)
Evian (France)	Naya (Canada)
Highland Spring (UK)	

Lowest mineral content
Poland Spring (USA)

How to use these tables

When you are choosing a mineral water, the same rules apply as to your general diet. If you are on a low-sodium (low-salt) diet, check the sodium content of the water first of all. An Australian study calculated that at around 300 mg per litre, drinking just 1.5 litres would be the equivalent of eating 1 g of table salt. Check nitrate levels (ideally the amount should be infinitesimal). And if you are using the water to prepare food for your baby, do not choose a high-mineral brand.

What are the health benefits of natural mineral water? An important one is that it can certainly provide more calcium than tap water. If you were drinking 2 litres per day of, say, Ballygowan, which contains 121 mg of calcium per litre, you would be getting around a quarter of your daily calcium requirement – especially important if you were dieting, were allergic to cow's milk or were trying to limit your consumption of dairy food (a rich source of calcium). The rest of your calcium requirement could be expected to come from spinach, oily fish, prawns, most nuts, sesame seeds – and chocolate! Even 2 litres of a lower-calcium water will still help very considerably, and once you have got into the water-drinking routine *you will be receiving that consistently every day.*

Moreover, although the matter is still under debate, there is growing scientific evidence that mineral water can genuinely alleviate certain health problems. For example, a recent study at the University of Cape Town in South Africa revealed that while high consumption of any kind of water limits the growth of kidney stones, the group of test volunteers who drank a high-calcium, high-magnesium mineral water (as against tap water) showed appreciably better results.

According to research carried out by the Free University of Berlin, mineral water that was low in salt but rich in sodium bicarbonate helped to lower blood pressure in a control group of older people. Experts at Wageningen Agricultural University in the Netherlands concentrated on magnesium – they had observed that low magnesium consumption led to heart problems in cattle and knew that it also played a role in human health. Trials with a human control group seemed to indicate:

a)   that magnesium was more readily absorbed through water than from foods;

b)   that 'when sport or exercise is advised to people who are at risk of heart disease, it involves consumption of high-energy foods, which generally contain much Mg (magnesium). Part of its effect could be obtained by drinking water with a high Mg content.'

The choice is yours, but I suggest you start with a water that is low in sodium chloride, balanced by calcium, magnesium and plenty of bicarbonates (those famous antacids that calm your digestion). Happy mineral-hunting.

FIZZICAL FACTS

I recommend drinking sparkling mineral water only very sparingly, and then choosing a low-gas water such as Badoit that comes from a naturally effervescent source (though even that is not quite as straightforward as it sounds). It is true that many people think still water is boring, but this book is about doing yourself good, and nothing I've learned about carbonated waters leads me to recommend them for your daily 2 litres.

We live in a society where fizz is prized. Champagne, lemonade, colas, so-called 'high-energy' drinks, premium lager beers – all of these are associated with fun and celebration. And so are sparkling waters, which are also often flavoured to make them even more 'interesting'. All these items are fine on occasion, but not as staple drinks. A short

only in violent cases.' Mineral salts and various fruit and sugar flavourings were later added, the beginnings of the modern soft drinks that remain modern society's favourite 'refreshers'.

And so here we are, in the twentieth century, with carbonated drinks of all kinds so dominant that when most of us think of 'refreshment' we think of 'fizz'. This is a pity, because in the USA – land of Coke and Pepsi and Dr Pepper – alarm bells are ringing about a generation of children who have grown up drinking highly sugared, artificially flavoured and above all carbonated American classics to the exclusion of natural water. A large number of children today are hyper-active (as a result, it is believed, of the excessive sugar content), overweight (from the unneeded calories) and there is evidence (including a recent US Department of Agriculture

....for your daily 2 litres, I recommend that you drink still water.

history lesson may begin to explain why. Ironically, artificially carbonated water developed from seventeenth-century attempts to imitate the popular and naturally effervescent waters of famous healing springs. By the 1770s Thomas Henry, a Manchester apothecary, was able to produce it in 12-gallon barrels, based on principles discovered by the famous chemists Priestley and Lavoisier. Soon Henry had many imitators, including an enterprising Swiss gentleman who moved his business to London and whose name is still world-famous. In 1794 he featured in correspondence from the engineer Matthew Boulton to the physician Erasmus Darwin (grandfather of Charles):

'J. Schweppe prepares his mineral waters of three sorts. No. 1 is for common drinking with your dinner. No. 2 is for nephritick patients, and No. 3 contains the most alkali given

report) that their bones may be dangerously soft. All this seems to have been unleashed by the carbonation process that Mr Henry and Mr Schweppes so innocently developed two hundred years ago for the dinner tables of the gentry. How could they have foreseen a world where millions drink nothing but carbonated liquids?

Unlike soft drinks, most artificially carbonated mineral waters have nothing added except carbon dioxide. But even here there are voices of caution. Respected nutritionist Patrick Holford is among these: 'Artificially carbonated water actually depletes our minerals ... the carbon in carbonated drinks is unattached and binds to minerals in us, taking them from the body. For this reason people who consume a lot of carbonated drinks have less dense bones than those who do not.'

I'm inclined to prefer things in their natural state. Plus I can't imagine downing a whole litre of gassy water in one! So for your daily two litres I recommend that you drink still water or, if you prefer, naturally sparkling mineral water. Treat a glass of carbonated water as you would a cup of coffee or a glass of wine. It is fine to choose fizz for fun and fashion.

'Natural' Fizz

Now for the waters which are allowed to describe themselves as 'naturally effervescent', such as Badoit, Perrier and Vichy Celestins (San Pellegrino, by the way, is artificially carbonated). Despite what you would expect, they are not, in fact, bottled exactly in the state in which they are found at source. The carbon dioxide naturally present in the water is extracted at this point and then restored at the bottling stage – without additional carbon dioxide being introduced. What is the purpose of this process and is it harmless? Inquiries to Badoit came up with the answer that it aims to ensure that impurities such as iron can be removed, though I was told there was nothing in writing that I could check which explained how it was done and why.

The FDA and the EU regulators are happy to allow the 'natural' description. Patrick Holford says approvingly that 'the carbon molecules in naturally carbonated water are bound to minerals found in the rock bed and deliver them into our bodies'. I'm still curious to know exatly how they recarbonate naturally effervescent waters, but if sparkling is what you crave, then these brands may be right for you as all or part of your daily two litres.

DOS AND DON'Ts FOR YOUR DAILY TWO LITRES

● **Do drink** natural mineral water whenever possible. It helps replenish vital minerals, cannot contain additives and must come from a safe, untainted source.

● **Don't be fooled** by labels which say 'table' water or 'natural' or 'pure'. Look for these words: <u>Natural Mineral Water</u> in the UK and Europe. And in the US, <u>Natural Mineral Water</u> or <u>Natural Spring Water</u>. Anything else may be no better than your own tap water – just more expensive.

● **Do examine** the labels of mineral waters and decide which brands contain the minerals you need for your optimum health. Avoid high nitrates and high sodium.

● **Do filter** tap water, if this is what you decide to drink. Point-of-entry ceramic and reverse osmosis filters are best. They counter bacteria and viruses as well as substance impurities. Carbon filters (the kind you can buy as part of a jug system) do a good job against substance impurities but not against organisms, and *must* be changed regularly or there is a risk of contamination.

● **Don't rely** on artificially carbonated waters for your essential daily intake. Naturally sparkling waters, often found at healing springs, are acceptable, but injecting artificial 'fizz' involves chemicals which are said to deplete the minerals in the food we eat and may cause loss of bone density.

● **Don't drink** distilled water – it robs the body of minerals (and usually tastes unpleasant) – or water that has been processed through a water softener (beneficial minerals may have been removed and replaced with sodium).

● **Do put** a jug of tap water in the fridge overnight to rid it of its chlorine taste but keep it away from any strong smelling food such as salad onions.

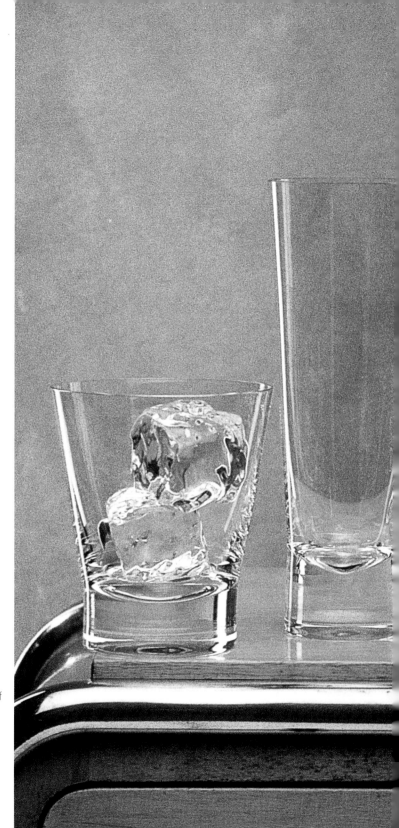

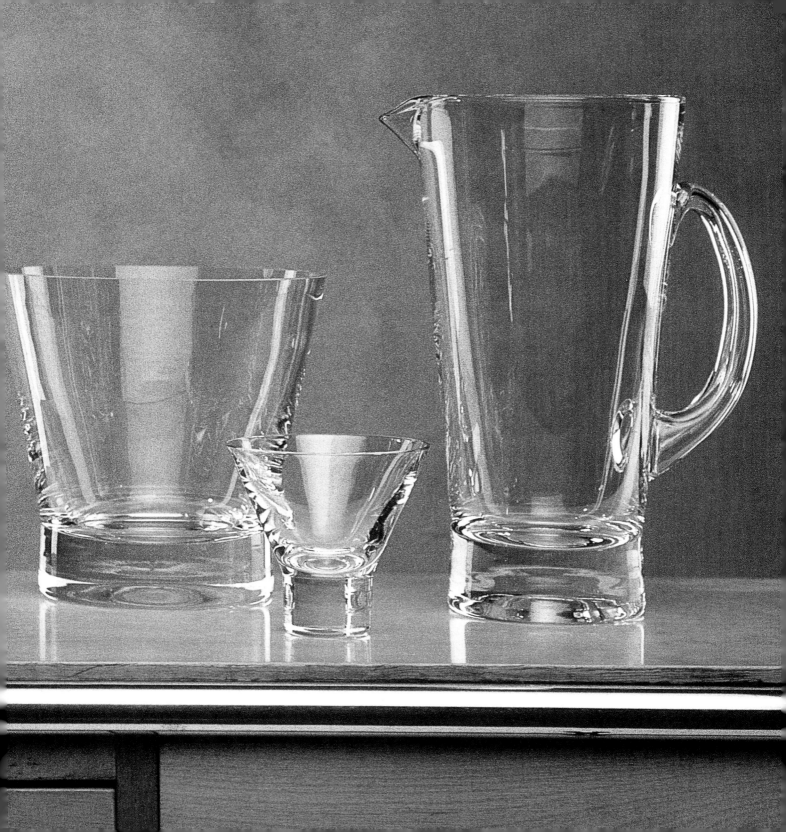

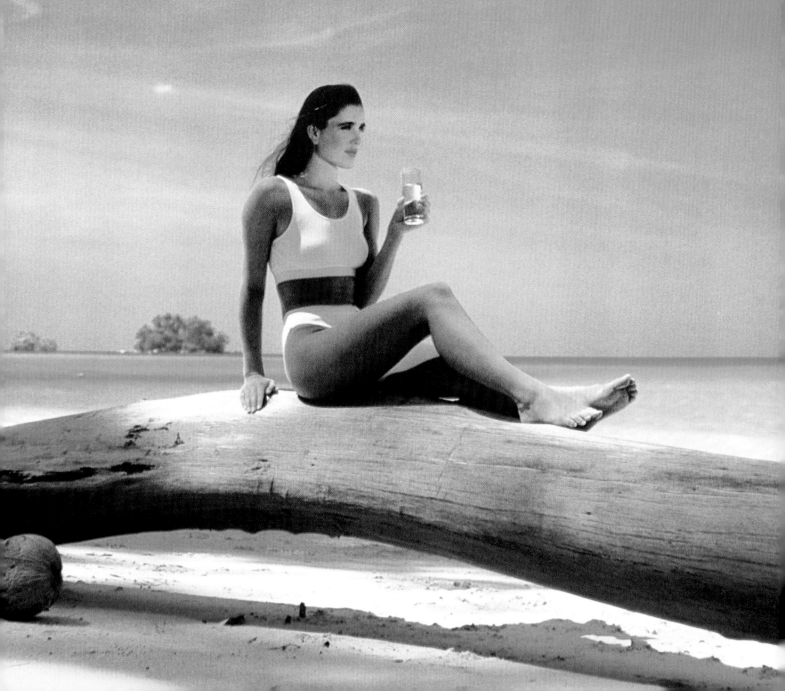

HYDROTHERAPY FOR HEALTH AND FITNESS

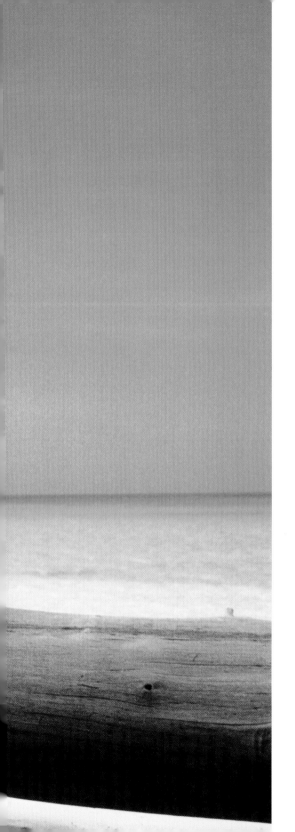

'She lays in the bath with the water touching
her all over, and remembered that not even
the most tender lover could do that. She wondered
if every molecule on the surface of her skin
was wet and what wet meant to such very
tiny matter. To make things worse, or at least
more difficult for the water, she raised her body
slightly, building an island chain of hip bones,
belly, breasts all of which began to dry at once.
She loved the water trails over her body curves,
the classical lines between wet and dry
making graph patterns which she thought might follow
the activity in her brain – all she wanted
was to be a good atlas, a bright school map
to shine up the world for everyone to see.

JO SHAPCOTT
FROM IN THE BATH

Hydrotherapy is something you're already doing every day. You have done it all your life. Hydro comes to us from an ancient Greek word meaning water. And from the moment you were born, water has bathed and benefited you. Here is a world of new and refreshing ways to treat every part of you. The term hydrotherapy embraces enjoyable, as well as rigorous, methods of watering your body from simple to sophisticated.

Thermal mineral waters, sea water, steam, jet-pressured hot and cold showers, baths of freshly drawn water, plain or in solution with marine algae, Epsom salts or essential oils – it's all part of hydrotherapy.

Hydrotherapy works because water itself is unique. Water does not irritate your skin. More things can dissolve in water than in any other substance. Water can transmit precious minerals to your body. And water has the unique ability to touch every part of you. The delight of bathing, showering and swimming comes from this ubiquitous sensation: plunge into water and suddenly it's everywhere! This is the day-in, day-out magic of pure therapy that water gives you.

A defining principle of hydrotherapy is the method of alternating hot and cold water to stimulate and rejuvenate the body. Even a splash of water can be quite a shock at first – breathtaking is another word for it. It is quite safe if you are reasonably fit. If you are the slightest bit worried about any method suggested, whether you are planning to try it at home or at a spa, first double check with your doctor as to its advisability, because whenever you are worried, your body cannot relax and the benefits of the treatment will be diminished.

You can learn to do many kinds of effective hydrotherapy at home, building on your daily shower and bath routine. Other methods require the skills of professionals. Steam

The delight of bathing, showering and swimming comes from this ubiquitous sensation: plunge into water and suddenly it's everywhere!

baths and sea-water treatments are two examples. Day spas can help you start or stay with a healthy regime, especially if you are low on willpower. (And who isn't.)

Visiting a residential spa could be your ideal holiday. Many spas are located at ancient sites where healing thermal waters have attracted people for centuries. Others are at pristine, ocean-side locations where thalassotherapy (sea-water therapy; see page 55) is offered. At spas, hydrotherapy is part of a total regime of treatments. Choose a spa carefully, according to your needs, your schedule and your budget.

When you arrive at a spa, you are usually assessed by qualified staff so that a programme can be designed to give you maximum benefit. Hydrotherapy at spas involves new and

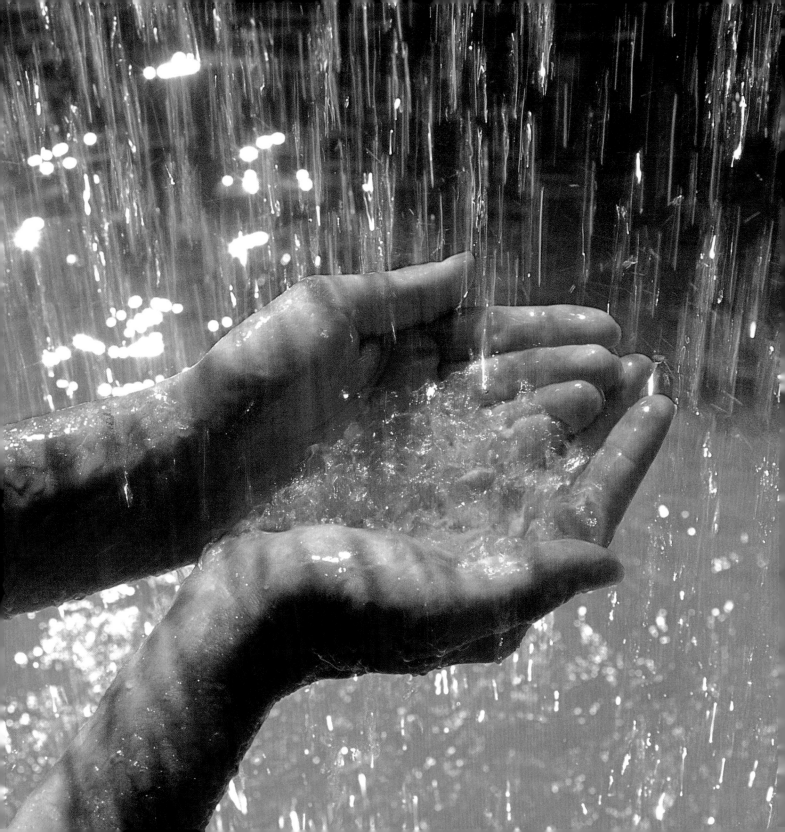

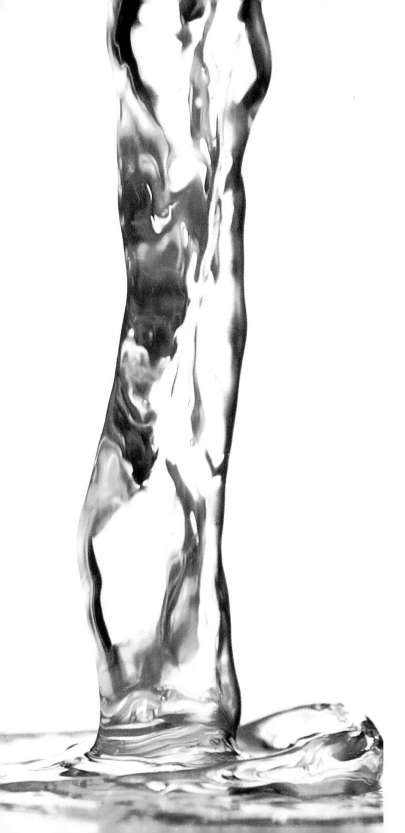

traditional treatments performed by professionally trained people. Depending on the spa, you will benefit from expert, hands-on massage as well as from high-tech machinery – like underwater jets aimed at particular parts of your body – sometimes simultaneously! Programmes lasting six days, with four treatments a day, are recommended for optimum results. Good spas offer specially equipped pools, gyms, whirlpools, steam rooms and plunge pools for total fitness and relaxation.

'Relaxation, however we achieve it, improves immune function and lessens arterial narrowing, two of the biggest factors that affect ageing,' explains Dr Michael Roizen, Professor of Internal Medicine at the University of Chicago School of Medicine. Roizen estimates that dealing with stress effectively can give you the vitality of someone *twenty* years younger. That in itself is reason enough to learn to water your body in new ways. In addition to reducing stress and anxiety, hydrotherapy helps you to sleep better; it eases muscle and joint pain; helps you recuperate from injuries; helps to replenish your stores of vitamins and trace minerals; stimulates your circulatory and lymphatic systems; lifts depression; improves overall skin tone; helps you slim; helps shift cellulite and helps your body flush out waste and toxins daily. Heal and rejuvenate yourself with the powerful, pure element of water by practising hydrotherapy at your own pace – at home and away.

HYDROTHERAPY'S HOLISTIC ORIGINS

Hydrotherapy was first made part of the practice of medicine over two thousand years ago by the Greek physician, Asclepiades. It was he who identified water as the key element of a total regime to counteract disease.

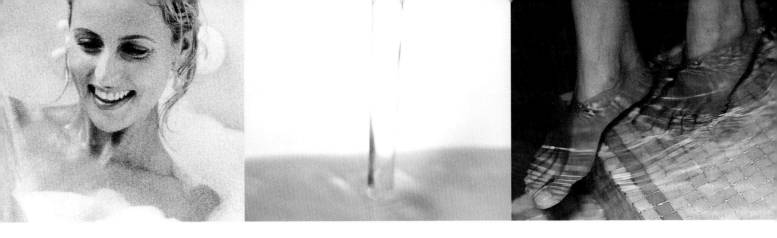

The history and myth surrounding this extraordinary man are as intertwined as the serpent coiled around a staff which is the ancient Greek symbol of the medical profession. Asclepiades was mortal, but, according to the poet Homer, had been taught medicine by the wise and kind centaur (half-man, half-horse) Chiron, who taught many young gods, including Achilles. In fact, such a wise and brilliant teacher was Chiron that Jupiter made Asclepiades into a star and placed him in the heavens as Sagittarius.

Asclepiades believed that the movement of atoms in the body caused disease and he advocated the therapeutic power of taking baths – along with following a proper diet and a regime of exercise and massage. Obviously this holistic approach worked and his reputation as a physician continued to grow into god-like proportions. Asclepiades came to be worshipped as a god, and a cult began in Thessaly and spread to many parts of Greece. He became so significant as a symbol of healing that later mythology records him as the son of the nymph Coronis and the great Apollo, god of music, prophecy, poetry – and healing.

It has taken us centuries to return to the holistic approach originated by Asclepiades. Make hydrotherapy part of your life. Combine it with a healthy diet, exercise and massage. No one thing ever works optimally on its own, not then and not now.

THE TOWN NAMED SPA

The word 'spa' has a wonderful, exhilarating sound to it, as if someone invented it to describe health and energy. In fact Spa is the name of a Belgian town amidst the Ardennes mountains which boasts several mineral springs popular for their beneficial effect for some two thousand years. Pouhon spring, in the town centre, is the most ancient. The Roman historian Pliny the Elder was the first to mention the springs, and for centuries people visited and made famous this site where you can still go and take the waters.

You can also do as the Romans did, without leaving home, by drinking the mineral water from this source. It is called Spa Reine and is available in the UK and continental Europe and on America's East Coast. Spa Reine claims to be the first bottled water ever to be exported, in fact to King Henri II of France.

'Spa' entered the language as the description for most natural springs, as well as for health resorts offering water therapy. Lately the term has been used to refer to everything from hair salons to nail-care emporiums, though ideally 'spa' should describe only places offering water therapy, including of course waterside resorts and clubs with swimming pools.

Tsar Peter the Great of Russia came to Spa in Belgium exhausted and suffering from 'dropsy', water retention in

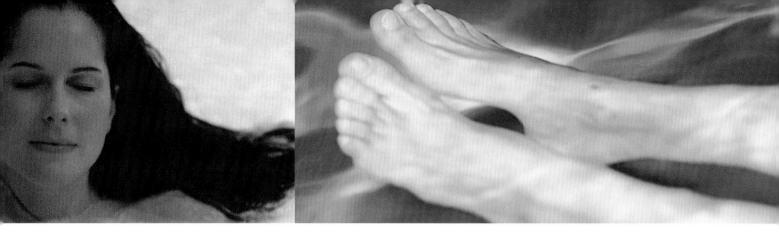

cavities and tissues of the body. He drank 2 litres (3½ pints) every morning from Pouhon spring and apparently recovered. Spa's status shot up, as did a statue of Peter the Great – who was over 2 metres (6ft 8in) tall! If you would like to return to the source and drink Spa Reine on site, you can stay in Spa and get slimming, anti-cellulite and organic peat treatments (the last is for rheumatism). For information see Directory (pages 152–4).

'TAKING THE WATERS' FOR HEALTH, FITNESS AND FUN

'Taking the waters' is the lyrical-sounding phrase probably invented by some early advertising genius to describe the rigorous regimes offered in the pioneering days of spas. It included bathing in the spa waters as well as drinking them, though not all spa waters were suitable for both forms of therapy.

Taking the waters at a spa could restore and relax you, treat and occasionally cure illness. This is true whether you visit a spa today or whether you were among 'the bibbers and bathers, the ramblers and gamblers, the sick and the sound', as one observer called the tens of thousands from all walks of life who flocked to spas in the eighteenth and nineteenth centuries. Three main factors – fashion, type of regime and

mineral content, determined how most people chose a spa. Similar reasons still apply.

Fashion

There were many who went to a particular spa simply because it was fashionable. Fashion is fickle, and grim or 'tyrant regimes', as they were known, were either in or out, often depending on where royalty were headed that year.

Visiting a spa held expectations of different things for different people, as it does today. Some people were ill and hoped to be cured. Others had less serious aches and pains. Most were more or less healthy and treated it as a social occasion. Some spas had casinos and other forms of entertainment. The origins of Derby Week, for example, can be traced back to horse-racing on the Downs at Epsom, one of the early British spas.

Travel itself was new and seen as therapeutic, so for many people spa-going became an annual social ritual of preventive medicine, as it is today. However, considering the rich foods and heavy drinking that characterised daily life in privileged circles in eighteenth- and nineteenth-century Britain and Europe, a week at a spa could not possibly make up for a year's partying, however strict the regime! Just as it cannot do now.

No Pain, No Gain

Some people chose which spa to attend on the basis of how grimly rigorous the regime was. The belief was that whatever the 'cure' involved, the more it hurt, the more it must work.

In terms of the strictness of the regimes, spas varied over the decades, swinging from one extreme to another, mirroring how people felt at the time about paying for the sins of overindulgence. Don't worry – spas are not as punishing they used to be, though Tyringham Clinic in Buckinghamshire is said to be quite tough. It reports an 87 per cent return rate, including one ninety-three-year-old who has been going there for thirty years! See Directory (pages 152–4) for more information.

The 'no pain, no gain' philosophy defined the early days of continental spas, and in Britain, Cheltenham Spa inherited

'Of all the uncomfortable ways of living sure an hydropathical cure is the worst: no reading by candlelight, no going near a fire, no tea, no coffee, perpetual wet sheet and cold bath and alternation from hot to cold.'

Cheltenham had become a rival to the long-famous spas at Bath and Tunbridge. Its rise had been sparked by the publication of Dr Short's *History of Mineral Waters* in 1740, in which the doctor claimed that Cheltenham's waters were 'the most effective in the country'.

How well did the 'no pain, no gain' regime work? Faith, a simple diet, plenty of drinking water and fresh air helped as much as the waters themselves to alleviate the ailments suffered by those in search of better health. Early spa visitors clearly found positive benefits for their gout, poor circulation, liver and various intestinal problems or they would not have

'Of all the uncomfortable ways of living sure an hydropathical cure is the worst: no reading by candlelight, no going near a fire, no tea, no coffee, perpetual wet sheet and cold bath and alternation from hot to cold.'

this philosophy. Just how strict was it at Cheltenham? Up at 4am, cold baths and a 16-km (10-mile) walk each day. The poet Tennyson gamely put up with this puritanical regime, which some called 'hydromania', at Cheltenham Spa for two months. This was the first English spa to be run on the principles of Vincent Priessnitz who defined key principles of hydrotherapy; he was not a doctor, but taught hundreds of doctors the virtues of his cold-water cures.

Fortunately, Tennyson had wit and patience. To a poet friend he wrote:

kept returning each year. But there is no conclusive evidence that even a strict regime cured those with serious illnesses.

The novelist Jane Austen, who suffered from a form of anaemia which attacks the adrenal glands, since known as Addison's disease, visited Cheltenham Spa. She may have decided to go there on the advice of her sister Cassandra, who had clearly enjoyed and benefited from Cheltenham:

'Dearest Cassandra, I am very glad you find so much to be satisfied with at Cheltenham. While the waters agree, everything else is trifling.'

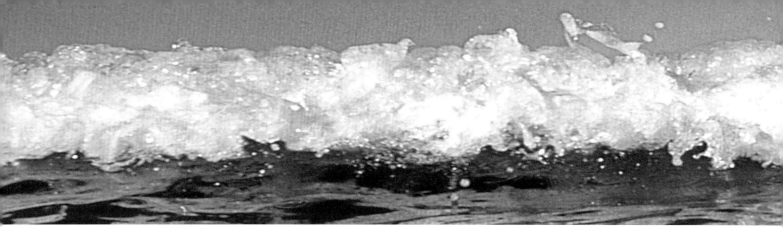

There is no record of Cassandra being ill; she may simply have wanted a restorative time. Jane, however, was probably well beyond a spa 'cure' no matter what the spa waters or the rigorous regime could offer. Sadly she died the following year.

Thermal spas at Bath in Britain, on the Continent and later on in New Zealand were very popular, though some people apparently overdid the thermal treatments and were more exhausted at the end of their stay than at the start. Effective, safe hydrotherapy, depended then, as now, largely on the water temperature: long, hot baths are not always best. Temperature plays as much a part in the healing and restorative process of bathing as does the water's mineral content. Dr Arthur Stanley Herbert, consulting balneologist to New Zealand and author of *The Hot Springs of New Zealand*, concluded that too much stress 'should not be laid on the mere chemical composition of a water'.

Mineral Content

Many people did choose a spa according to the water's mineral composition. It sounds sensible, but it was as much guesswork as chemistry that informed doctors' and patients' decisions about which minerals could cure specific illnesses. It would take pages to list the promised benefits from each spa, and contradictions abounded.

Wiesbaden, near Frankfurt, was one of Germany's most famous thermal spas visited by over 15,000 people annually in the nineteenth century chiefly for medicinal reasons. The main spring, Kochbrunnen (the scalding spring), has many mystical qualities attributed to it. Salt and lime are its main mineral constituents.

In 1839, a Dr Richter published a list of countless 'disorders' which Wiesbaden waters would help, whether taken internally or externally.

These included such uncomfortable conditions as: ...acidities, furred tongue, loss of appetite, sense of tightness or oppression about the stomach and bowels after food, liver congestion, haemorrhoids and kidney problems, gout, rheumatism, and paralytic affections occasioned by the poisons of lead, arsenic, mercury, or contusions of the head and back'. Dr Richter also noted that 'the Weisbaden waters (like many other mineral springs) are lauded as efficacious in certain complaints and defects of both sexes, which it is not convenient or proper to notice in this place'.

There was great debate then and now as to the nature and degree of the mineral content needed to benefit, no less 'cure', various conditions. Many problems that people brought to the spas could be eased whatever the mineral content simply because the spa regime itself provided a

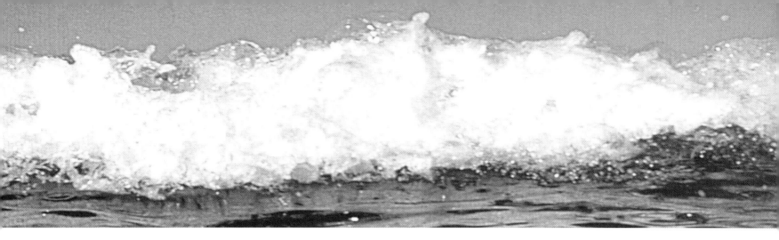

simpler diet, fresh air, pure water and a restful break in outdoor surroundings – a healthy contrast to their usual day-to-day life.

Thalassotherapy

The energy of the sea can move boulders. Think what it can do for your mind and body.. Thalassotherapy spas are increasingly popular and seaweed itself is the latest buzzword in beauty treatments. The term thalassotherapy was coined in 1869 from the Greek 'thalassa', meaning sea. It describes the systematic use of sea water, seaweed, sea mud and beach sand to benefit health. In the 1870s the French biologist René Quinton recognised a similarity between the mineral composition of sea water and our own blood plasma, and concluded that contact with sea water must be restorative. Indeed the ancient Greeks and Romans were convinced of its curative effects, and valued it highly.

The theory is that we are able to absorb vital minerals through our skin from sea water by immersing ourselves in it. Today, orthodox opinion is divided as to the degree of nutrients absorbed, though the successful use of skin patches (such as nicotine patches for people attempting to give up smoking) suggests that the skin may be far more adept at absorption than many experts believe.

Dr Christian Jost, medical consultant at Ireland's Inchydoney Thalassotherapy Centre, attributes the following health benefits to the minerals found in sea water: calcium and magnesium are excellent for rheumatism and osteoporosis; sodium and potassium are excellent for the muscles; sulphur for vascularisation (the development of blood vessels); selenium for energising the cells; nickel for the regulation of carbohydrates; zinc for immune defence; aluminium for anxiety; iodine for fat metabolism. Heating the sea water helps the minerals penetrate the skin. According to Dr Jost: 'Twenty minutes in a heated thalassotherapy pool will ensure that your essential store of vitamins and minerals are fully replenished.

Before joining the Inchydoney Centre, Dr Jost was a sports injury specialist and he continues treating this sort of problem at the Centre. In common with many thalassotherapy practitioners he believes that the combination of the body's buoyancy in sea water, together with the water's rich mineral content, makes thalassotherapy particularly effective in healing muscle and joint injuries.

Individual thalasso treatments are said to boost your circulation, tone and relax you, reduce cellulite, relieve aching muscles, help you recuperate from injuries and alleviate stress. Post-natal programmes, offered in several French thalassotherapy centres, help mothers rest and relax with their new babies and restore their body tone.

The beneficial effect of thalassotherapy is also endorsed by Dr Rajendra Sharma, medical director of Forest Mere, one of Britain's premier spas, which offers an inland version of thalassotherapy with its heated sea-water pool. Dr Sharma spans both the alternative and mainstream medical worlds, and sees the process of hydrotherapy itself, especially sea-water treatments, as highly therapeutic, whatever the degree of mineral absorption.

A true thalassotherapy spa, according to the French Fédération de Mer & Santé, must use fresh (sometimes called live) sea water, has to be located on an unpolluted beach and has to operate under medical supervision. You should look for all three when booking into a thalassotherapy spa to get the full benefit.

Inchydoney is the only true thalassotherapy centre in the British Isles. You will be spoiled for choice in Europe, especially in France, and in the Caribbean. The best travel agency to help you locate a spa for you is Erna Low (see pages 152–4).

Ideally you should spend six days at a spa, with four treatments a day, though a weekend is a good start. For example, at Ireland's ocean-front Inchydoney Thalassotherapy Centre, two luxurious days will cost you £250 and include six key treatments: *balneotherapy* – heated sea-water baths for hydromassage; *hydrojet* –sea-water jet massaging to increase circulation; *algotherapy* – heated body wrap in marine algae to aid circulation, cleanse skin; *brumisation* – inhaling energising ionised sea water mist; *cryotherapy* – cold sea water leg-wrap with marine algae to boost circulation and reduce water retention; *massage* – to relax you or to relieve pain.

Forest Mere in Hampshire boasts a new salt-water hydro pool and has excellent treatments and facilities. While it is not true thalassotherapy because it is inland, and not all the elements are present, it is situated on a beautiful lake and you will get a good idea of the effectiveness of certain aspects of thalassotherapy. While you are there, try another form of hydrotherapy: swimming! You can learn to swim or improve your technique. Take private swimming lessons for £17.50 a half-hour. Then, when you do go to the beach, you can enjoy it more fully. Forest Mere offers a special short break of three full days with a two-night stay, starting at £300 for a single room (economy). This includes two full body massages; one facial; one eastern scalp massage; one thalassotherapy hydro pool session; unlimited use of all facilities including sauna and steam room; complete exercise/relaxation programme; and three meals a day.

Marine-based beauty treatments are offered at day spas in cities too: for example, Villa Thalgo day spa in Paris. Seaweed- and marine-based beauty products are big news now, and you can buy wonderful concoctions for your own home spa. Always read the labels before you buy, however: not every product with a seafaring name contains enough marine elements to make it any different from an ordinary enjoyable aquamarine foambath.

Purists take baths in Thalgo, which is 100 per cent pure natural micronised marine algae. It certainly smells authentic – like the seaweed it is – though you can counteract its low-tide tang by adding a few drops of pure lavender oil to the water. Seaweed purifies the ocean and acts similarly to detox your body if used religiously. Before you part with nearly £20 for a box of ten Thalgo sachets, prepare for your bath water to turn mocha brown. You could instead opt for Elemis Cellutox

Herbal Bath Synergy, which blends algae and essential oils, has a lemon scent and promises similar detoxifying or 'body-cleansing' benefits.

MAKE HYDROTHERAPY WORK FOR YOU

I find it is helpful to combine at-home hydrotherapy methods with those at a day or residential spa. This way, you can ask questions and get personal advice from experts, then carry on at home with confidence throughout the year.

Your body changes each day, each month, over the years, and with your way of life. Try not to be too set in your ways. Think of how you change your hair and make-up and the clothes you wear, according not only to fashion, but, more importantly, to what makes *you* feel good. Hydrotherapy is no different. Fortunately, water is as fluid as life itself and can adapt to suit you.

Generally speaking, you will achieve the best results if you follow a holistic approach, just as the god-like Greek founder of hydrotherapy advised. Use various forms of water therapy, from bathing and showering to professional treatments, in combination with a sensible diet, a regime of regular exercise and massage.

The glossary of terms on pages 88–9 summarises the language of the various types of hydrotherapy treatment and can be used for quick reference, particularly when you are considering which day or residential spa you might like to try.

There are now thousands of spas to choose from around the world, with day spas in most big towns and cities. I have concentrated on spas which provide water therapy. To get you started, I have selected those which are the most highly recommended. An easy way to explore the tantalising world of spas is to visit the following website: www.spafinders.com.

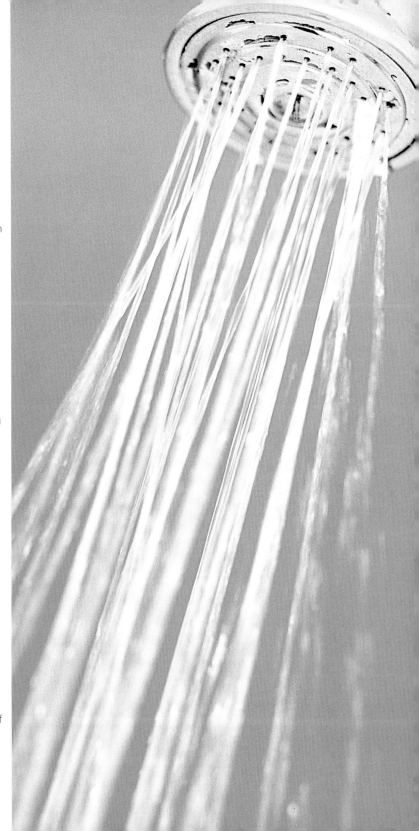

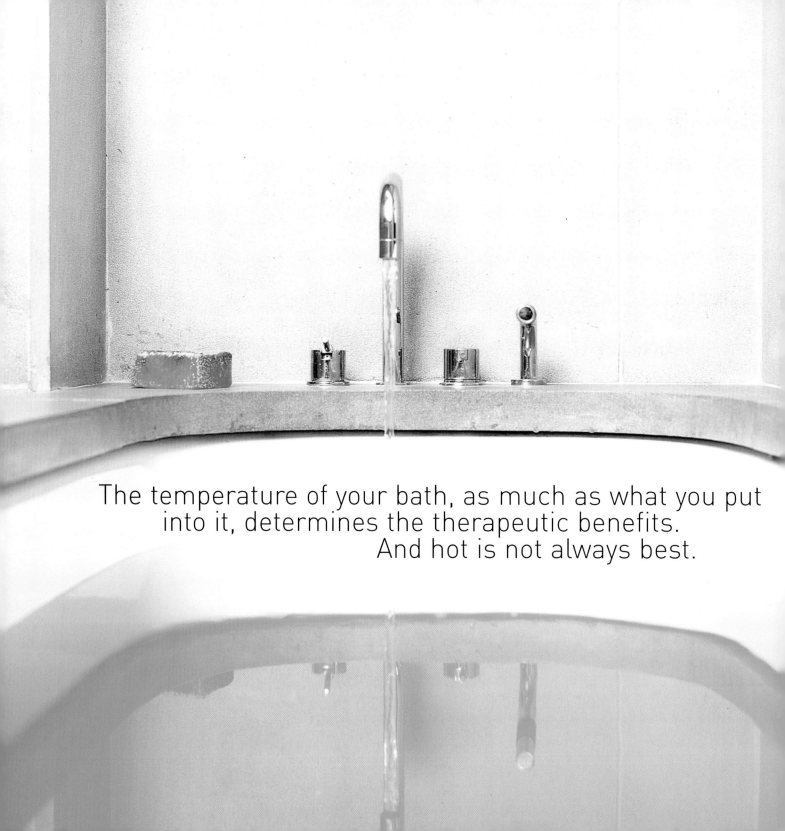

The temperature of your bath, as much as what you put into it, determines the therapeutic benefits. And hot is not always best.

Before you book into any spa, ask lots of questions!

What you do every day to maintain your health and well-being is as important as all the invigorating visits to day or residential spas, however special. First, learn how to make the most of your own bathroom 'spa' and enjoy hydrotherapy at home.

AT-HOME HYDROTHERAPY:
DON'T GET INTO HOT WATER

A hot bath spells luxury and relaxation for most people, especially in winter. No one I know would voluntarily sink into a cold, or even cool bath at the end of a long day. Nor would I have ever willingly stood under a cold shower after my hot one! While there are excellent reasons to take hot baths, there are also reasons not to make your daily bath too hot – and very good reasons to follow hot with cold.

The temperature of your bath, as much as what you put into it, determines the therapeutic benefits. And hot is not always best. Only by understanding how different parts of your body react to hot and cold water will you know how and when to take the most therapeutic bath or shower.

Here is one example which might ring true for you, and begins to explain how hydrotherapy works. I used to take a hot bath when I had a headache, thinking that it would relax the tension and relieve my pounding head. Usually, at the tail end of the working day, around 7 pm, I would sink into as hot a bath as I could stand. The heat of the bath, my headache and the lateness of the hour made me sleepy enough to want only to lie down afterwards, which I would do. Invariably my headache would worsen into a full-blown migraine, so that even if I did manage to drop off to sleep, I would wake up half an hour later with a now-crashing headache and a dry mouth, far too nauseous to eat dinner and altogether more tense.

Where was I going wrong? Hot water does relax your muscles and relieves stiffness, but it also expands your blood vessels. The heat makes the blood rush to your head, which it is doing anyway when you have a headache. By lying down immediately after the bath, I was allowing congestion to build up in the very areas that were already in trouble: neck and head. If I had been able to have a massage to alleviate that tension, it might have helped slightly, but not sufficiently to offset the effect of the very hot water expanding my blood vessels.

Now when I have a headache I take a lukewarm bath, with an ice-cold compress on my forehead, for about ten minutes. The bath relaxes me and the ice gives me a feeling of instant relief, almost numbing the headache. Importantly, it constricts the blood vessels. Also, when I lie down to relax afterwards, I make sure my feet are warm.

Headache or not, a long, hot bath (longer than five minutes and hotter than body temperature) is not generally a good idea. It depresses your circulation as well as your metabolism. Taking a bath that is over five minutes long and hotter than 104°F or 40°C tends to exhaust you. This explains why a very hot bath first thing in the morning will work against your body's natural rhythms. Instead of helping your body gather its energy for the day ahead, it will deplete you. It also dries out your skin by drawing out your body's natural oils. My own solution in the morning is to shower. But if you love to bathe in the morning, take a warm or 'neutral' bath, (at body temperature). This can be deeply relaxing and is the principle behind 'flotation' – minus the Epsom salts.

Whether you shower or bathe, finish off with a shower of cold water. If you can't take the shock – I promise, it gets easier – try sponging yourself all over with cold water. Cold water stimulates your circulation, closes your pores, tones and invigorates you. Why? Cold water warms you up by causing your body to produce the opposite reaction. Recent research shows that a two- or three-minute cold shower every morning strengthens the immune system and reduces your chance of infection – backing up pioneer hydrotherapist Father Kneipp's cold-water therapy of a hundred years ago. Enjoy the healthy kick of cold water, and always wrap up in a thick towel afterwards.

CONTRAST-HYDROTHERAPY GIVES YOU ENERGY

If you have been able to follow your warm shower or bath with an exhilarating splash of cold water, or indeed have managed to give yourself a quick finishing shower of cold water, you are ready for this next step, called contrast-hydrotherapy. It's very easy to do at home, but it does take a bit of willpower! Leslie Kenton, the inspiring and well-known health and beauty writer, swears by this method. She uses it often and finds it 'energy-enhancing' and 'energy-balancing', giving you energy if you are feeling low, as well as calming you when you are stressed.

There are significant benefits attributed to contrast-hydrotherapy. Author Helene Silver, founder of the Inner Beauty Institute in Sausalito, California, considers it one of the most invigorating showers you can take and believes that it stimulates all the body functions, especially the glandular system. It revitalises your skin and improves circulation. It works according to one of the most basic principles of hydrotherapy, which is to contrast hot water with cold. But rather than just sponging off with cold water after a warm bath or shower, you alternate hot water with cold several times in rapid succession and for longer periods. I find that it is much easier to accomplish all this in the shower, though you can also do it using the bath and shower.

First of all, whether you are at home or at a spa, make sure the room is warm. You should not feel chilled at any point. Nor should you try this if you are feeling chilled yourself to begin with, for whatever reason. (As with any method using extremes of temperature, check first with your doctor if in any doubt. Do not use this method if you suffer from high blood pressure, a nervous disorder, or any kind of organic disease, or if you are very weak or have insulin-dependent diabetes.) Have ready a large, thick towel and a terry towelling bathrobe.

Take a hot shower, or bath, for two to three minutes. Follow it with a shower of cold water lasting twenty seconds. Repeat this procedure three times. Always remember to begin the contrast method with hot water and to finish with – you guessed it – cold! That's where the willpower comes in. As you get used to the contrast in temperature, you can extend the hot shower (or bath) to four minutes, and the cold shower for as long as one minute. The point of the cold water is to constrict the blood vessels, and even twenty seconds has been shown to be sufficient – so don't worry if you cannot manage the cold interval for longer than twenty seconds. It still has a beneficial effect.

If you think this contrast-hydrotherapy method is too rigorous, consider yourself lucky that you were not at the Gräfenberg spa started by one of the pioneers of hydrotherapy, Vincent Priessnitz. He believed that health was the body's natural condition and was convinced of

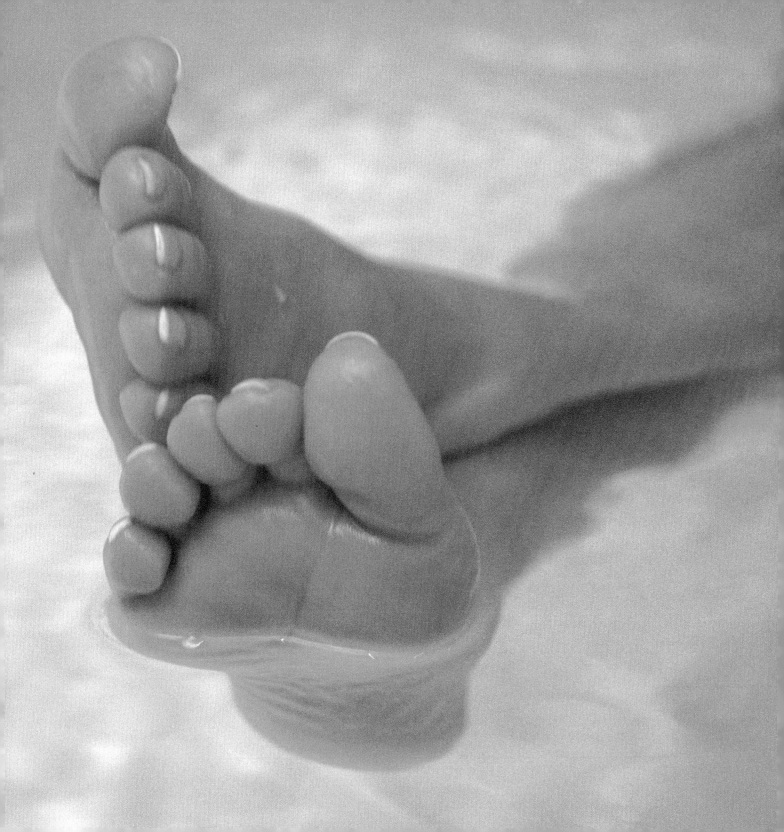

water's healing powers. The body could restore itself if all toxins and poisons were expelled. His techniques included drinking twelve glasses of water a day, a diet of coarse bread and milk, and a very untantalising schedule of treatments at his spa! Patients had to lie with their heads in cold basins of water, have water sprayed up their genitals and lie wrapped like mummies in wet bandages for hours. Finally, from a height of 6m (20ft), icy water was released on the lot of them! As Roy Porter details in his history of medicine, *The Greatest Benefit to Mankind*, all this went down a treat 'on an overfed, overdrugged and stressed-out generation'. In 1839 the spa boasted among its visitors a monarch, a duke, a duchess, twenty-two princes and 149 counts and countesses.

it this way in his excellent book, *Hydrotherapy*: 'Certain parts of the body, when heated or cooled, will have reflex effects on the circulation of distant areas…. The skin of feet and hands is reflexively connected with the circulation to the head, chest and pelvic regions (especially the bladder and reproductive organs, including the prostate in men).'

The nineteenth-century pioneer of hydrotherapy, Father Sebastian Kneipp, was a great advocate of cold-water therapy, believing that it boosted the immune system. And recent research results at London's Brompton Hospital have confirmed this.

Kneipp also believed in the effectiveness of alternating hot and cold water, for body and foot baths. Foot baths had been a feature of water therapy since Greek and Roman times, and

If your feet feel good, so does the rest of you.
Your feet control how the rest of you feels.

WET YOUR FEET WITH FATHER KNEIPP

If your feet feel good, so does the rest of you. Your feet control how the rest of you feels. When they are cold and wet you are probably uncomfortable; if your shoes pinch, your face shows it; when your feet are warm and dry, the rest of you relaxes.

Reflexology is based on the principle that massaging and manipulating different parts of the foot has a positive affect on your organs and circulatory system, improving your energy and generally clearing blockages. Hydrotherapy also works on the reflexive principle. For example, by soaking your feet in hot or cold water, or by adding certain ingredients to your foot bath, you will be treating other parts of your body because of the reflex connection between them and your feet.

Osteopath, naturopath and author Leon Chaitow explains

Kneipp brought to this ancient pleasurable treatment his own holistic approach treating thousands upon thousands of people in German spas, several of which still use his name for the treatments which follow his techniques.

Here are two excellent ways to bathe your feet, one using contrast-hydrotherapy, the other adding mustard to hot water. Both are very easy to do.

Father Kneipp's Foot Bath

Try this whenever you are feeling congested or generally sluggish. It is meant to help clear your system by stimulating circulation of the blood and lymphatic system and is a treatment for colds, sinusitis and headaches.

Unlike your arterial blood, which is pumped around your

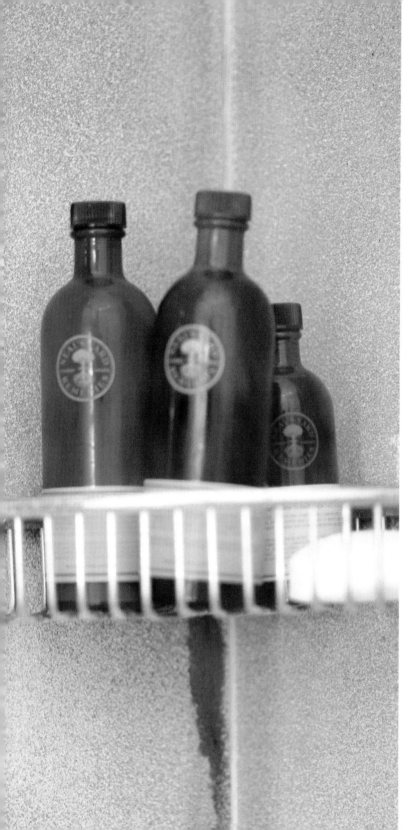

body by the heart, the lymphatic system is fairly stationary unless you do something to get it moving – with exercise, massage, skin brushing or contrast-hydrotherapy such as this foot bath. The sensation of 'heavy legs', which describes the sluggish, weighted-down feeling that comes from bad circulation, sitting too much and simply from the effect of gravity, can be helped with this treatment. You will see professional spa treatments offered for helping 'heavy legs', especially at thalassotherapy centres. This would be a good way to maintain the benefits of that treatment.

To prepare the footbath take two buckets (or tubs), each one big enough for both your feet to fit in comfortably. Fill one with hot water and the other with cold, both to a depth well above your ankles. Sit in a chair and place your feet in the hot water bucket for three to five minutes, then switch to the cold tub for thirty seconds. Do this twice.

Pass the Mustard

This foot bath also stimulates your circulation and helps rid your entire body of toxins and waste, according to Helene Silver. She comments: 'Miraculously, mustard foot soaks have been used successfully to relieve the pain of earache, tooth abscess and sinusitis by drawing the body fluids to the surface of the feet.'

To prepare the footbath find a bucket or tub you can stand in and fill it with very hot water – as hot as you can take it. Dissolve three tablespoons of mustard powder in the water (don't use more than three tablespoons because mustard is powerful) and bathe your feet in it for twenty minutes. Your skin will redden as the mustard starts to act, dilating the blood vessels near the skin's surface, bringing fresh blood to the area and also drawing lymph to the surface. This is what

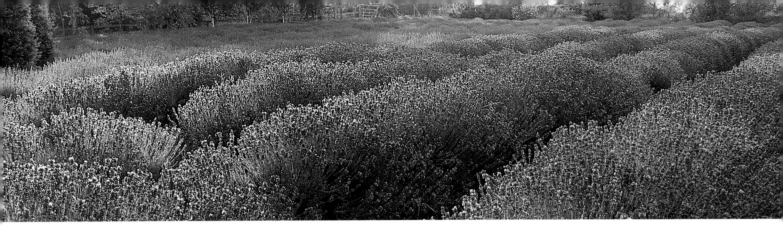

helps your body flush out the toxins and waste, making the mustard foot bath a good treatment whenever you want to detox your entire system.

he lost much of his work! Fortunately, he left us two massive encyclopaedias, one on science, the other on medicine. This became the key medical source of the Middle Ages.

lavender works to clear your head, lift your spirits and relax you.

AROMA-HYDROTHERAPY: BATHING IN FRAGRANT WATERS

You can do a lot more for yourself than to add synthetic detergent to your bath: this is what many bath preparations contain. Why not use natural fragrant essential oils from plants to heal and revitalise you with aromatherapy? Flowers, herbs and leaves have been used for thousands of years for pleasurable, preservative and medicinal purposes. Bathe in your favourite naturally scented essences, at home, to your heart's delight.

Distilling the pure essential oils from plants dates from the Middle Ages, and we have Avicenna, the great Arab philosopher-physician to thank for this. He was the genius-son of a Persian tax collector and by the age of sixteen was already practising medicine. An extraordinary scholar, he wrote 270 works, many on horseback, so the story goes, in between journeys and military campaigns, and unsurprisingly

The world of aromatherapy is yours to discover simply by visiting a health store or pharmacy. By all means check out which oils are meant to treat the condition you wish to alleviate or create the mood you wish to achieve. Also, just follow your nose! If you love a scent, find out what it is meant to do. Your sense of smell could be telling you something important – I loved the scent of lavender before I learned that it works to clear your head, lift your spirits and relax you. See the following page for a quick summary of the benefits attributed to each essential oil. Use one essence at a time to benefit from its full impact. Then, as you get to know which oils do what, you can experiment and mix them. (Use them for massage too.) You need only a few drops. Essential oils will stay fresher longer if you keep the bottles tightly closed and store them in a cool, dark place.

Don't make your bath too hot, and relax for half an hour in the fragrant waters.

ESSENTIAL OIL	PROPERTIES
BASIL	Fresh invigorating oil, good for clearing the mind and aiding concentration, especially when tired. Ideal after a stressful day.
CHAMOMILE	Excellent for skin care, especially sensitive and problem skin. Soothing and relaxing, encourages sleep. Ideal for stiff joints and muscles.
CYPRESS	Natural deodorant and astringent often used in aftershave. Useful for combating cellulite and sweaty feet. Useful during menopause.
EUCALYPTUS	Strong antiseptic. Burn to reduce airborne germs or add to massage oil for a clearing chest rub. Ideal for sportspeople.
GERANIUM	A refreshing balancing oil for mind and body. Good in times of confusion. Excellent for skin care.
JUNIPER	Antiseptic and astringent ideal for oily skin. Add to massage oil for combating cellulite. Massage into scalp to encourage healthy hair. Has a cleansing effect on the body.
LAVENDER	Mildest but most effective of all essential oils. Can be used neat as an antiseptic. Excellent for skin care. Restive in small amounts – helps restore balance and encourages sleep.
LEMON	Excellent antiseptic. Refreshing and uplifting – useful insect repellent and hair rinse. Can be used to lighten dull stained hands or to tone and condition nails and cuticles. Blends well with other oils.
MARJORAM	Warm, comforting oil. Useful for tired muscles and ideal after sports – simply add to massage oil and use as a rub. Massage abdomen during menstruation. Encourages sleep.
NEROLI	Calming and soothing during times of stress, helps restore sleep. Ideal for skin care, especially mature/dry skin.
PEPPERMINT	Clearing, penetrating odour. Invigorating – ideal travel companion. Use to bathe tired sweaty feet. A good insect repellent. Has a cooling effect on the body. Ideal for use by sportspeople. Best not used on children under three.
ROSE	Widely used in skin care, especially for dry, sensitive skins. Soothes anger and grief. Renowned sensual properties.
ROSEMARY	One of the most stimulating of all oils. An ideal pick-me-up, aids memory and clear thinking. Use to combat fatigue and clear a stuffy atmosphere. A useful hair tonic and muscle rub. Ideal for sportspeople.
SANDALWOOD	Often burnt as an aid to meditation. Creates an exotic atmosphere, excellent for skin care, especially when dry or sensitive. Useful for dry or damaged hair and as a body fragrance. Antiseptic, soothing.
YLANG-YLANG	A sweet, exotic oil, long used for its sensual properties. Soothing and relaxing during times of tension. Ideal for dry skin and as a hair rinse.

Information reproduced by kind permission of Kobashi (see Directory pages 152–4)

THE ELATION OF FLOTATION

Flotation, developed during the Second World War, is a brilliant method of hydrotherapy which aims at total relaxation. It involves floating in water in utter darkness with no external distractions. You don't have to know how to swim, because you will be floating in an extremely salty solution which keeps you buoyant and totally relaxed. Most importantly, the water has to be kept at body temperature. You can go out for a float or simulate the experience at home.

Away

What happens if you go out for a float? You will be shown into a room which has in it a flotation tank (ideally in a spa setting). This is usually body-sized and specially designed to keep the water heated. You slide or climb into the tank and the person in charge gently closes the top portion over you. It is dark – rather like entering a drawer of salty water. This can feel quite claustrophobic at first.

The room itself should be comfortably warm so that you do not get a chill when you emerge, two hours later. As you come out, blinking, into the daylight you feel tremendous elation. Even people who were previously blasé about flotation admit to this feeling once they have tried it.

Dr John Lilly, who developed the technique, found that lying in a body-temperature bath, combined with sensory deprivation, not only produced a deeply relaxing effect, but was also very effective against anxiety, depression, tiredness and even high blood pressure.

At home

A variation of flotation you can try at home is a 'neutral' bath without salts. You simply bathe in plain water at body temperature. You will not be as buoyant, but it is still very relaxing and extremely beneficial, lifting depression and calming you.

Salts or no salts, make sure your bathroom is warm, so that the water stays at the same body temperature. Keeping it at a consistent temperature is not all that easy and this is one of the disadvantages of home flotation. You will have to top up a bit with hot water from time to time, to ensure that it stays at 'neutral'. A bath thermometer may be helpful. Because you will be floating for a long time (up to two hours), you may be tempted to make the water too hot but it's very important to avoid doing this. You will be in your own environment, so you will be relaxed throughout the float which is the aim of the procedure.

If you want to try home flotation with salts, you will need 450 g (1lb) of Epsom salts. If you like, you can add 250 g (8 oz) sea salt (not table salt) plus a teaspoon of iodine (use the clear kind or it will stain the bath). These additions make it as similar as possible to a sea mineral water bath. You should relax in the bath, which should be full and not hotter than 40°C for twenty minutes. Epsom salts are very stimulating and twenty minutes is sufficient at home. Wear an eye mask so that you will not be tempted to read. Do not soap yourself – this is not an activity bath – and do not shower afterwards. Just towel yourself dry, stay warm and head straight for bed.

Epsom salts will make you sweat a lot, so don't forget to keep drinking water handy by your bedside. This is a perfect detox bath: once a month is all you need.

If you prefer *not* to sweat and detox, as described above, a 'neutral' bath is the better choice. Anyone with a serious cardiac condition or diabetes, or who has any broken skin, should not take the salt bath.

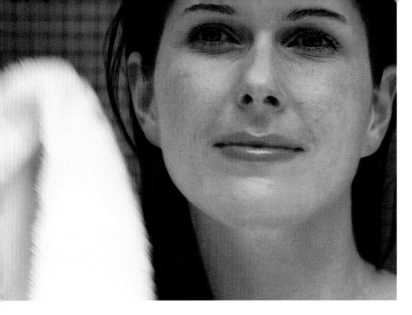

passages, so try some slow, deep breathing while you relax in this bath. Rosemary oil also works as a decongestant. It is meant to stimulate the nervous system and ease rheumatic aches and pains. Both eucalyptus and rosemary are antiseptic, so these are healing oils for minor skin problems – eucalyptus is good for chapped skin. Sandalwood oil cleanses and moisturises the skin. In India, its scent is used to induce a meditative state. Plan to spend twenty minutes in this deep heat bath. It should unwind you into a relaxed state.

TAKE A SITZ & SIT MORE COMFORTABLY

Sitz is German for seat, and sitting in the bath (as opposed to lying or wallowing in it) can be very therapeutic for certain extremely irritating conditions such as cystitis and haemorrhoids. If you can take the cold, there is also a sitz bath designed to stimulate your kidneys and reproductive organs – perhaps even your love life.

APRES-EXERCISE BATH

This is a very good after-exercise bath which uses deep heat together with essential oils to help relax your muscles. It is especially welcome on damp, cool days and in the dead of winter. And it is worth doing even if your only exercise has

You should not follow this bath with a cold splash: simply towel dry vigorously, put on warm clothes and relax.

been sitting at a computer, pushing a pencil or standing for long hours in one position.

You should not follow this bath with a cold splash: simply towel dry vigorously, put on warm clothes and relax.

First, make sure the bathroom is comfortably warm. Keep the door closed to retain the steam from the heat of the bath. Pour the following essential oils into a hot (but not scalding) bath: 10 drops each of eucalyptus and rosemary; 5 drops of sandalwood. Eucalyptus oil helps ease aching joints and muscles, and its vapour is useful in clearing your respiratory

At spas with special sitz (or hip) baths it is easy to arrange contrasting-temperature sitz baths in which your bottom sits in hot water, for example, while your feet are placed in cold.

Sitz baths designed with two separate compartments also enable you to benefit from alternating-temperature baths where the water is quickly changed – bottom in hot, feet in cold, and then vice versa.

Contrasting- and alternating-temperature sitz baths can be very healing, but they are fairly tricky things to organise at home, although not impossible.

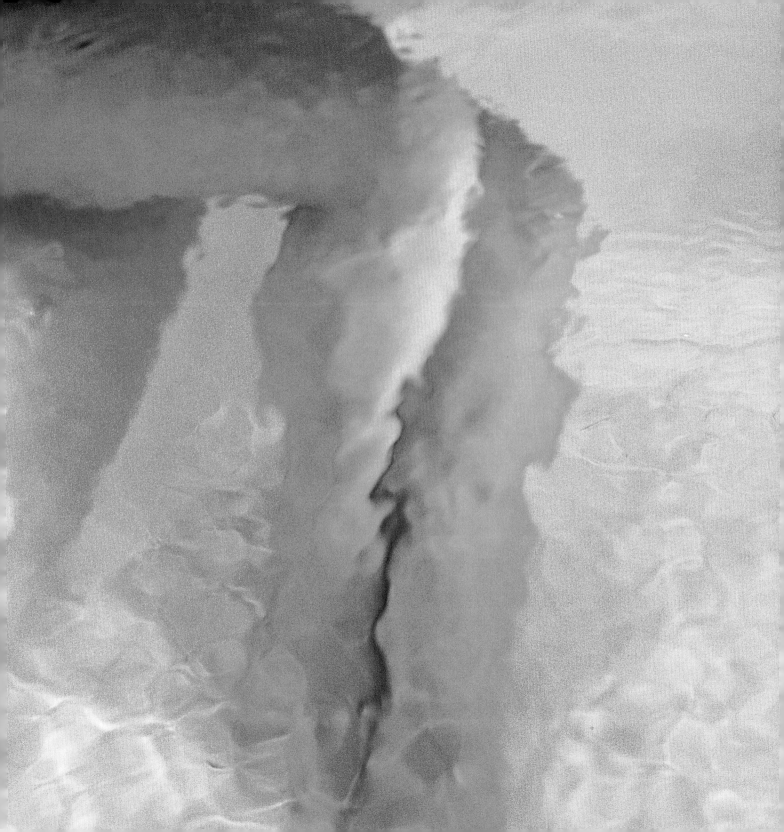

My view is that you should aim to do the best you can at home and leave it to the professionals to give you the specialist hydrotherapy treatments at a spa. So I am suggesting only single-temperature sitz baths here, each of which you can do easily and well in your normal-length bath. See which one suits your needs and take a sitz!

The 'Neutral' Sitz Bath

This bath is said to be helpful for cystitis sufferers. Simply half fill the bath with water at body temperature. Sit down in it with your knees bent and drawn toward you so that they are out of the water and your feet are in the water. Bathe for half an hour.

and stimulate your kidneys and reproductive organs. Some call it a youth bath, perhaps because it helps to be young when it comes to the cold bit!

As with any treatment involving cold water, you should only do this if you are in good health. You must be warm to start with and your bathroom should be cozy, too. Choose a medium-sized towel to drape over your shoulders or wear a T-shirt.

Fill your bath with 20 cm (8 in) of cold water straight from the tap and –this is the hard part – just sit down in it. The towel or T-shirt will keep the top half of you warm. Raise your feet so that they are out of the water. You can rest them on the edge of the bath or prop them up on an inverted bowl.

Sitz baths designed with two separate compartments enable you to benefit from alternating-temperature baths where the water is quickly changed – bottom in hot, feet in cold, and then vice versa.

The Hot Sitz Bath

This is meant to speed the healing of haemorrhoids. Half-fill the bath with hot water (106–110°F or 41–43°C) and sit down in it, knees bent and drawn toward you so they are out of the water (as above) for up to ten minutes. Following your bath, apply a flannel or small towel wrung out in cold water to the affected area, then dry gently.

The Stimulating Sitz Bath

Remember how cold showers were meant to dampen the ardour of young men? Well, they got it all wrong. Cold water is actually very stimulating. This bath is said to rejuvenate you

Stay in for one whole minute. Counting helps keep your mind off the cold. Saying out loud, slowly and rhythmically, 'One and two and etc.' will help you breathe steadily and give you the equivalent timing for each second. (Otherwise, wear a waterproof watch!)

At first you will feel cold, and then warm. When you get out, quickly rub yourself dry, get into something comfortable and head for bed.

Proponents of this method promise that you will grow accustomed to the cold. When you do, you can gradually increase the cold sitz bath to two minutes' duration and then to three.

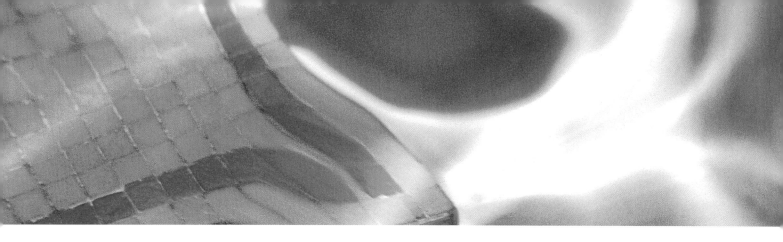

GIVE YOUR BATHROOM THE SPA TREATMENT

This section is designed to help you to create your own ideal environment for your daily at-home hydrotherapy. It is all to do with feeling utterly relaxed as you lie in your bath – rather than anxiously staring up at a peeling bathroom ceiling wondering how you will ever find the time or money to fix it.

You may already have the perfect bathroom. If so, enjoy and make the most of it. Also, take note of what it is that makes your bathroom ideal: is it modern, traditional, colourful or calm? This can help you choose a spa which suits your personality. You might want a similar environment or long for the opposite.

Whenever you return from a holiday during which you have enjoyed spending time in a particularly well designed bathroom it gives you a fresh outlook on your own. Fortunately, a bathroom is usually the smallest room in the house. Even small changes can make a big difference and need not cost the earth. Light, air, warmth, privacy and easy maintenance are the five essential elements to consider if you are going to enjoy and benefit from at-home hydrotherapy. See which of these aspects needs addressing in your bathroom. Did I mention water? Of course, it helps if everything works to begin with: the best water pressure

possible, plentiful supplies of hot water, and drains that drain. Fancy taps and towels are icing on the cake. First sort out the basic plumbing.

LIGHT AND AIR

These elements are best looked at together. A light and airy space is a healthy environment, and bathrooms are no exception. Damp, dark bathrooms with insufficient ventilation will never feel or be invigorating. They could also encourage germs to breed. Don't worry about how much moisture you create in your bathroom but remember that the constant build-up of steam means that you need to let fresh air circulate year round. If you have a window, make sure you open it. Fling it wide open in spring, summer and autumn and let in as much fresh air as possible in winter. Otherwise a permanently damp atmosphere will pervade the room and encourage the growth of unhealthy mould.

Many en-suite bathrooms, as well as those in city flats and apartments, rely on vents for air circulation, electrically operated or otherwise. Make sure the vent is working properly. If the filter is one you can remove and clean, or replace, remember to do this on a regular basis. If you have an air-conditioner, don't forget to do the same, and keep it unclogged.

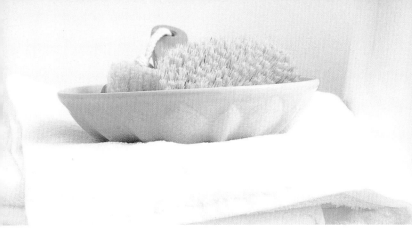
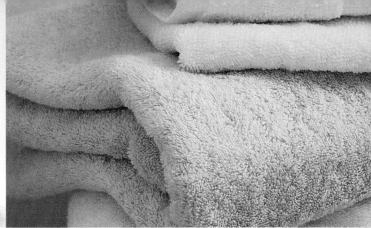

Good bathroom lighting is as necessary as daylight. If your bathroom has no window to provide natural daylight, you really do need to get the lighting right. Try halogen rather than tungsten bulbs for a fresh, white clean light. Or mix the two to get the best of both if you have more than one light source. Here is my ABC of lighting for the ideal bathroom:

Ambient lighting This should be on a dimmer switch so that you can wake up to a 'sunny' bathroom even in pre-dawn

and deepens circles under your eyes. It is neither efficient nor cheerful, especially in the morning.

Candlelight This is wonderful to bathe in. Put a simple candle sconce or two at mid-height on the wall. Also choose a fat, long-lasting candle to place by the bath. Match the scent to your mood, or to the fragrance of the essential oils you are bathing in to intensify the therapeutic effect. Keep to naturally scented candles or use unscented ones. Beeswax

wake up to a 'sunny' bathroom even in pre-dawn winter gloom

winter gloom, and relax with low-level soft light at night. Some dimmer switches hum annoyingly, especially at low light levels. If you want to bathe in peace, install the switch outside the bathroom door.

Bright directional lighting Design this to surround your mirror, movie-star style. A semi-circle of small, opaque bulbs gives you the ideal light conditions for putting on make-up, tweezing your eyebrows and any other close-up grooming activities, such as putting in (or searching for) contact lenses. Directional lighting adds to ambient lighting. Depending on the size and shape of your room, you could put both sources on one dimmer switch. Whatever you do, don't settle for a single overhead light – it casts uneven shadows

candles are beautifully subtle and last a long time.

Warmth

Heat is as necessary as fresh air to fight a damp atmosphere. Install whatever type of device gives you a steady, controllable source of heat so that even without a stitch on, you don't feel chilly. If your bathroom is cold, you will never attempt anything but a too-hot shower or bath and you won't really relax.

Warmth is also achieved with colour. Do you like your bathroom's colour scheme? Once the room is physically warm, you can experiment with the whole spectrum of hot, warm or cool colours. You probably already know which colours calm you and which ones invigorate. I'm drawn to

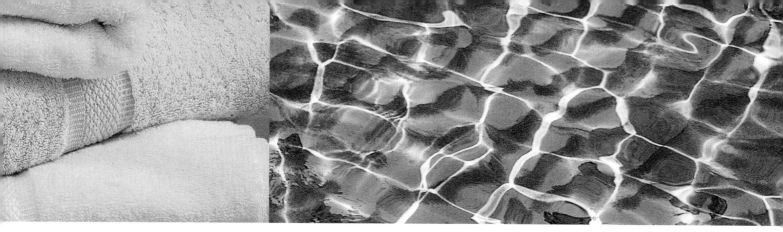

blues and aquamarines. Choose the decor according to what colours make you feel good.

Privacy

A good door is not the only thing you need to give you this essential element while you are in the bathroom. If you have windows, you will probably need to screen yourself from public view while still allowing in daylight. Shutters with adjustable louvres are a classic solution. Another idea which combines light and privacy comes from Alison White, who *Elle Decoration* magazine describes as a 'window-covering design specialist'. She recently developed a simple cotton roller blind which lets in light at the top but is dense at the bottom (See Directory pages 152–4.)

Sound creates privacy too. A radio, cassette or CD player in the bathroom allows you to be in your own space, detached from the activity in the rest of the house. Bach soothes me. For relaxing music and sounds inspired by the sea listen to Dolphin Dreams, (Northsound Series; CD available on the internet through Amazon.com).

Easy Maintenance:

Bathrooms are 'wet' areas in the language of spa design, changing rooms are 'wet and dry' and relaxing rooms are 'dry'. Apply this to your own house and you will see that while your living room or bedroom might be suitable for wallpaper and carpets, your bathroom is probably better with painted walls and tiled floors. Hard surfaces are so much easier to maintain, and if you're not worried about maintenance, you are much more likely to be relaxed in the bathroom. You can choose from real slate, limestone and beautiful terracotta tiles for the floor, as well as from many convincing imitations, though since it is a small space, you might be tempted to go for the real thing if that's your heart's desire. Give your tiled floor a once-over mop and it's clean as a whistle however wet it gets. Wood is excellent too, but seal it well. Otherwise, like carpet, wood can remain damp, retain smells and needs more scrubbing to get it clean.

Painted walls are hard-wearing, especially in a damp atmosphere, and simple to change if you get bored. Magazines and books are bursting with ideas. Kevin McCloud's *The Complete Decorator* gives you the whole story on natural paint and decorating techniques. You might like to stencil a wave, shell or dolphin theme on your walls. To learn how, read Lyn Le Grice's classic book, *The Art of Stencilling*. Lyn's wealth of experience in designing spas enables her to help you with imaginative yet practical solutions for your spa bathroom. (See Directory pages 152–4 for contact details.)

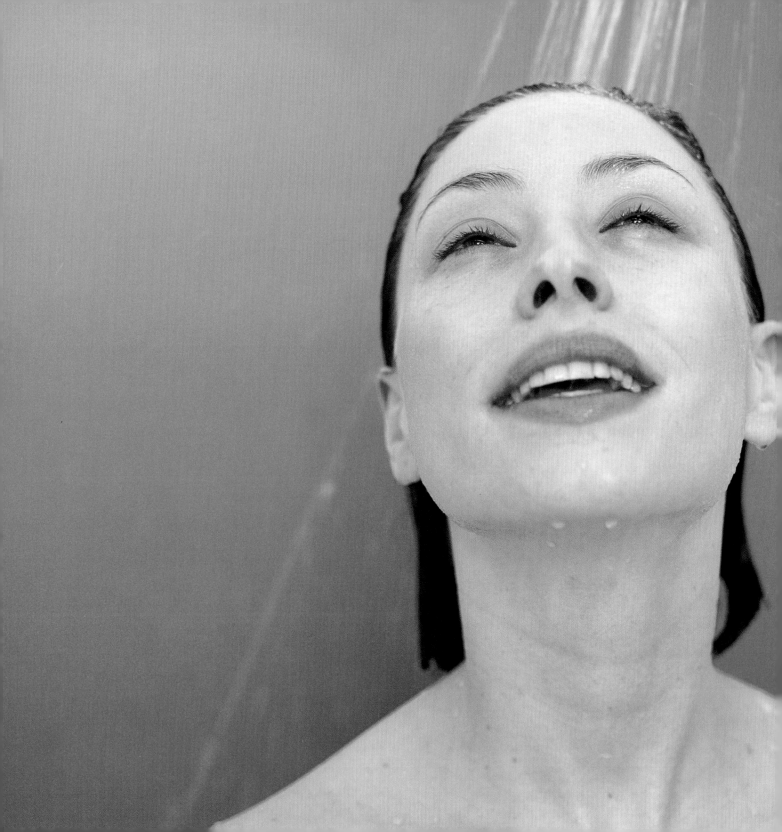

BATHING BEAUTIES TO UPGRADE YOUR BATHROOM and YOU

Here is a top-to-toe tour of the essential hardware and software designed to turn your bathroom into an invigorating spa so you can indulge in pure therapy.

The Hardware

If you are about to upgrade your bathroom or add a new one, you're spoiled for choice. Basins, wcs and baths range from the stark elegance of Philippe Starck's latest designs to the romance of antique cast iron and copper. A late nineteenth-century copper bath will set you back £6,500. After that, almost anything seems reasonable! You need a bath and a shower. Depending on your budget, you could install a Jacuzzi bath, and a multi-spray shower enclosure with overhead, hand-held, mid-body and foot sprays all in one unit. The shower would enable you to water-massage every millimetre, and the bath would provide treatment and a treat. If you like antique baths, you can reclaim one or buy a reproduction. Aston-Matthews boast the widest range in Britain. (See pages 152–4.)

The Software

Thick and thirsty towels, stacks of pure glycerine soaps, a natural sponge and a strong, long-bristled body brush are easy ways give your bathroom spa-like splendour. Pure white towels look wonderful and can keep their freshness for years because it is so easy to wash them at high temperature. Droyt's soap is a clear favourite – 10 per cent pure glycerine and all natural oils: palm, castor and coconut. Droyt's was first developed in Russia in 1907, is still made to the same recipe and is cut by hand into all shapes and sizes. The Body Shop, in most major cities, is a good source of bath and shower treats.

More serious software

A good way of deciding how serious a spa is about therapy is noting which products are used there. You may want to bring items from these top treatment brands home: Aveda, Clarins, Clinique, Decleor, Dermalogica, Elemis, Espa, Ionithermie, La Prairie, Phytomer, Repêchage, Thalgo, Thalocéan. Some spas are 'one-brand spas', using, for example, only Clarins, or Thalgo. Others, like Bliss in New York, have developed their own brands. Day spas in major department stores like Harrods offer you treatments using several different brands.

If you are willing and able to spend a little more (in some cases a lot more), you can pick from a range of highly specific solutions for your body which contain special (some call them 'signature') ingredients aimed at treating particular problems. Consider their claims carefully. Usually the phrase 'helps to' prefaces each claim, because nothing can work miracles though repeated use of a good product can improve your body. Remember that no product is effective unless you use it regularly as part of a total regime of healthy eating, exercise and hydrotherapy. It is up to you to decide whether a product is worth the money. Claims include 'helping to' firm flabby skin tone, reduce cellulite, rehydrate skin to delay the ageing process, increase circulation to eliminate toxins, and alleviate joint and muscle aches. Promises to relax you are easily kept, as are exfoliating and skin polishing.

Experience the more expensive delights by trying them at a day spa. There, the professional staff will be using them properly; then you can follow on at home. That's how I found my current favourites: Dermalogica's Hydro-Active Mineral Salts, their Streamlining Body Toner, and Thalgo's Micronized Marine Algae.

FINDING A SPA TO SUIT YOUR NEEDS

Here are six ways to find a day spa that's right for you. You can also use this guide to find a residential spa. What is the difference? In some cases there is none – they are one and the same place. Spending a day at a residential spa is a great way to it test out to discover whether you would like a longer stay in the future.

For example, if you spent a day at a top-of-the-range, fully equipped, mainly residential spa, you would benefit from free use of a gym with instructors on hand at all times, a sauna, steam room, whirlpool or Jacuzzi, swimming pool, plus a selection of specific body and facial treatments, with massages lasting a minimum of forty minutes. At the other

an extensive menu of individual treatments using many different products, from Decleor to Elemis, La Prairie and Thalgo. Try a Thalgo Body Wrap to reduce cellulite (£50), or book in for your Ultimate Day of Beauty (£350). This includes Deluxe Body Polishing, Hydrotherapy Underwater Massage, Soothing Body Wrap and Massage, Light Champagne Lunch, Deluxe Manicure, Spa Pedicure, Luxury Facial, and Shampoo, Cut and Dry. Harrods salon is on the fifth floor of the store.

At Harvey Nichols in London you will find the Aveda Concept Salon, and perhaps Kate Moss. Aveda products are mainly for face and hair rather than body. Still, this salon offers a Hydrotherm Massage, a full body massage during which you lie on a warm-water cushion like a waterbed, so

Here are six ways to find a day spa that's right for you. You can also use this guide to find a residential spa. What is the difference?

end of the scale you can spend a day at an expanded health and beauty salon which offers excellent body and facial treatments, but with no pool or gym. Decide what you need according to your physical and emotional needs, schedule and budget. I have listed six ways to help you find the day (and residential) spa that's right for you with examples in each category. Additional spa suggestions follow this section.

1. Check into good department stores

Department stores have expanded their hair and beauty salons, so although you will not find swimming pools or gyms, you can benefit from excellent body and face treatments worth a visit lasting from an hour to a day.

At Harrods in London for example, you can choose from

that heat transmits itself to you evenly. It is very relaxing, takes an hour and costs £65. The salon also offers a one-hour anti-cellulite detox treatment using a seaweed wrap (£48).

Harvey Nichols in Leeds also offers a day-long total experience at Aveda's Urban Retreat for £160. This includes a body and scalp massage, facial with massage, manicure and pedicure, shampoo and blow-dry, and make-up touch-up.

2. Seek out the best hotels

Hotels do not always welcome non-residents into their spas but you have nothing to lose by asking, wherever you live. In London, Claridges, the Berkeley Hotel and the Dorchester each has a welcoming spa well worth a visit.

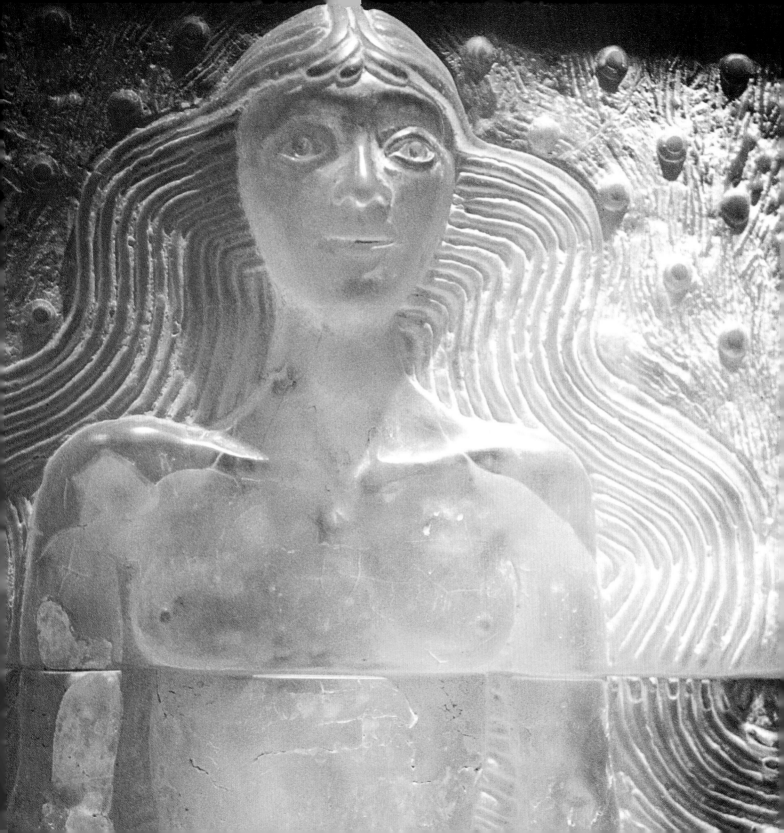

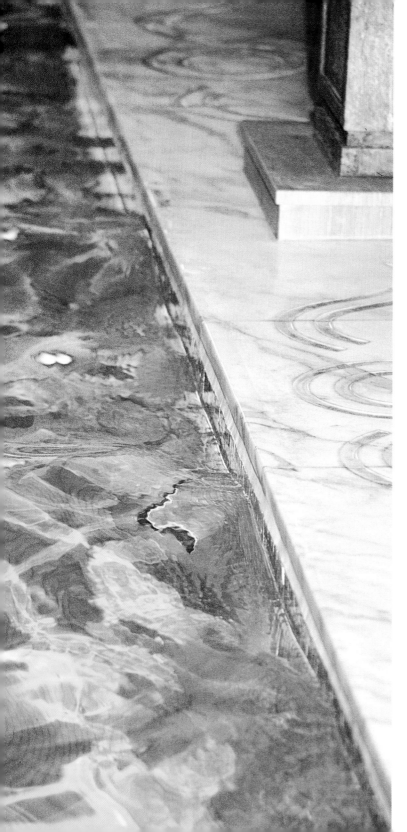

Claridges boasts the Olympus Suite, a small, peaceful spa/gym. There you can enjoy an Espa Restorative Mud Envelopment which aims to replenish your body's store of minerals (£60). If you have the time, try the Stress Recovery Day, Detoxifying Spa Day or Fitness Revival Day. Each offers you various treatments, all using Espa. Including lunch, these days cost £150. Espa mineral salts are green and gorgeous and make an invigorating at-home spa treatment. A jar (£16) is enough for fifteen baths.

If you like open-air pools, spend the day at the Berkeley Health Club and Spa. It has a roll-away roof for sunny days, and you could find yourself sunbathing next to Brad Pitt or Gwyneth Paltrow. The pool is heavenly. This elegant spa uses only Christian Dior products for facials, body scrubs and treatments. There is also a gym, plus sauna and steam room. Packages cost from £75.

The Dorchester offers a Thalgo Spa Day for £175. This includes a complete series of hydrotherapy treatments including hot and cold contrast jets-showers to boost your circulation, a hydrotherapy bath to tone specific areas and help lymph drainage, a body scrub for exfoliation and detox, a full body massage, a facial and use of sauna, Jacuzzi and steam room. Everything is immaculate, and lunch is included. You can also book individual treatments.

Urban spas outside big cities might be less expensive, but are they good value? The following examples offer real value for money. Use them as a benchmark for a hotel spa near you. Or take a weekend break.

Cardiff's five-star St David's Hotel charges £98 for an Espa Stress Recovery Day and includes use of the hydrotherapy pool with reconstituted sea water, three treatments lasting three hours, one of which is in a hydrotherapy bath and uses detoxifying purified seaweed; a body massage and facial; time to relax in the 'sanarium' – a cross between a sauna and a steam room – and use of the pool and gym. A two-course lunch is included.

In Edinburgh, the Balmoral Hotel offers you a Total Luxury Day at £115, which includes a seventy-five-minute full-body aromatherapy massage, a seventy-five-minute facial, manicure, pedicure and lunch. There is a fully equipped gym with instructors, aerobics room, pool and steam room. Salon manager Lyn Jones recommends steam after massage 'because it helps to relax the muscles...we don't think you achieve the same effect if you have to rush out after a relaxing treatment'. Agreed.

Spa-finder Stan Cooper of Healthy Venues can help you short-circuit the search for your nearest day spa in Britain, usually within an hour of where you live and his booking service is free. No matter which spa you visit, a Pamper Day costs £99, £10 more at weekends. Pamper days are held mostly in hotels and represent good value rather than top-end luxury. You can enjoy relaxing beauty and body treatments and usually hydrotherapy (there is a pool at all but two of Healthy Venue's portfolio of day spas). A Pamper Day offers a full body massage, facial, manicure, pedicure, and use of sauna, steam room, and swimming pool. A light lunch is included. Healthy Venues also handles arrangements for residential spas in the UK.

It has a roll-away roof for sunny days, and you could find yourself sunbathing next to Brad Pitt or Gwyneth Paltrow

3. Consult the consultants

Most spas, both in the UK and abroad, will welcome you on a day-only basis. You might live near a spa and would like to try it, or plan to travel abroad and would like to experience a day or two at a particular spa. Erna Low has for thirty years specialised in arranging tailor-made residential spa holidays outside the UK, particularly at thermal and sea-water spas, and is also happy to be contacted for day spa arrangements. The company handles spa bookings in seventeen countries, including France, Spain, Italy, Austria, Switzerland, Hungary, the Czech Republic, Germany, Malta, Madeira, Portugal, Sweden, Finland, Israel, Cyprus, Ireland and South Africa. Last-minute bookings are 'a speciality'. There is no fee for this knowledgeable consultant and booking service.

4. Go surfing or by the book

Spa Finder USA is a magazine with an extensive database on the web where you can find information on residential day spas. Most spas offer individual treatments and/or day packages. Spa Finder specialises in locations in the USA, but it also covers some European spas, as well as a few in more remote places.

Have fun surfing on www.spafinders.com.

Spa Magazine is a Seattle-based quarterly magazine providing information on spas all over the world. It is available on subscription only (tel: 00 1 206 789-6506 for details), but you can also access information by clicking onto www.spamagazine.com

Fodor's guide *Healthy Escapes* can help you find spas in

the USA, Canada and the Caribbean. It makes excellent bathtime reading, even if you never set foot outside the door. You can find it at bookshops or by telephoning + 44 (0) 279 973-9790.

5. Find a healthy friend

This option is a bit cheeky, but if you have a friend who belongs to a health club, why not ask to go as his or her guest for the day! Most health clubs are for members only (for two great exceptions, see below). Guests' fees are usually nominal – £10 gets you in as a guest to any of the hundred or so Livingwell Clubs across Britain, including Brindleyplace in Birmingham, with its gorgeous pool and state-of-the-art gym,

welcome to enjoy its deluxe facilities on a day -spa basis. If you book into one of the many day packages, you have full use of the 25-m (27-yd) swimming pool, Jacuzzi, state of the art gym with cardiovascular and weights machines, full-size exercise studio, steam, sauna and relaxation rooms. The atmosphere is decidedly relaxing (not dizzy disco) and beautiful. Marble, slate, mahogany and mosaic will make you feel very spoiled. Soothing aromatherapy scents waft through the club, and head of spa Libby Eley emphasises the club's holistic approach to relaxing your mind, body and spirit. A Detox Day, for example, costs £110. You can choose what best suits you after a consultation. It typically includes a seventy-five-minute body wrap treatment using Elemis or Aveda,

Pamper days are held mostly in hotels and represent good value rather than top-end luxury.

steam room, excellent treatments and canal-side brasserie. You must be accompanied by the member, and usually you cannot be a guest at any club more than a few times.

This is a good way of seeing whether joining a club is right for you. For information on joining Livingwell Clubs telephone 0800-136-6363. Their stand-alone clubs (as opposed to those in hotels) are often best, though obviously as a guest you cannot be too choosy!

6. Go Clubbing

The two top London health clubs described below are open to non-members on a day-spa basis. See if the club you would most like to join offers a similar package.

The Club at County Hall is said to be the first twenty-four-hour health club in London. As a non-member you are

a G5 massage to stimulate circulation in hips and thighs, and a facial, reflexology or scalp massage.

Champneys Piccadilly is a great escape in the centre of London and, again, you do not have to be a club member to enjoy it. Champneys set the UK standard for health spas a long time ago. Staying there is extremely expensive, as is club membership. This day spa alternative offers a package of very good value treatments and relaxation for heaps less money. The Top-to-Toe package includes a body massage, a Decleor facial, a pedicure and manicure, and your choice of body scrub, make-up or sun-bed session. There is a swimming pool, spa bath and steam rooms. 'We like to think that when you step into Champneys Piccadilly, you leave life's irritations behind you,' says Jo Plane, events and marketing co-ordinator. To see if it works for you, book your away day.

DEDICATED DAY SPAS IN FIVE STRESSED-OUT CITIES:

London

The Grove offers a totally integrated approach to staying healthy and looking good. It is currently London's only spa and gym to include a complementary health clinic. Since its opening in 1997, diners at Kensington Place, the popular restaurant opposite, must be thinking twice about ordering more wine or tucking into dessert.

The Grove's holistic approach is not against life's little pleasures, but it does take your body's shape seriously. Medical doctors well versed in alternative health will discuss various treatments with you to help determine what you need from the huge menu. You can benefit from five separate but interrelated aspects: Complementary Health Therapies, Total Body Spa, Personal (one-on-one) Training Gym, Fertility and Pregnancy Care Clinic, and Detox and Weight Control Clinic. The full six-week Detox Programme has apparently yielded impressive results. Max Tomlinson, naturopath at The Grove, tailors it to you and your schedule. Make a start with a Detoxifying Body Mask (£50) to encourage the elimination of toxins and prepare your body for a course of treatments. If you can spare only half an hour, the 'fairly deep' Phytomer Thalassotherapy massage will introduce you to the combined benefits of seaweed, California stretching, shiatsu, lymphatic drainage and Swedish massage, all for £40.

New York

The Soho Sanctuary is a laid-back place dedicated to de-stressing you. It's about beauty and relaxation achieved through massage and mud therapy rather than hydrotherapy or thalassotherapy. There is no pool or gym and none of it comes cheap, but to many it is the best day spa in town. Choose from the extensive menu of individual treatments if the Day Package looks likely to over-stress your bank balance.

A body mud wrap using mineral rich Moor Spa costs $145. If you would also like a thirty-minute massage, add $45 and, for a facial, another $35. The Day Package includes aromatherapy with massage, scalp massage, back facial, reflexology and two-hour facial, as well as lunch. Plan on spending five and a half hours and parting with just over $500.

Bliss set the pace in New York for day spas. Some find it too buzzy, but most people love it. There is a hydrotherapy bath for $55 with active seaweed and oils; or try the Fully Loaded Facial which includes an acid peel, oxygen wrap, collagen ampoules and a seaweed mask for $185. New Yorkers are demanding, so expect the treatments at NY day spas to be top notch – if they are not, act like a New Yorker and complain. This place can make you feel good even if you just read their catalogue!

Visit their website at www.blissworld.com and order from their tempting range of own brand and leading-brand products for yourself, or go on site to Soho and 'bliss out'. Appointments are notoriously hard to get here so plan ahead. (Note: Bliss in London is not connected with this spa).

The Repêchage Spa at The Galleria on New York's East Side offers you a quick way to beat jet lag with city-based thalassotherapy. You lie in a tank while alternating jets of warm and cool sea water massage your body. A mist of seaweed wafts over you throughout. This Vita Cura Treatment aims to oxygenate your blood by stimulating your circulation. A revitalising thirty-minute treatment costs $75. Since it's tricky to time an appointment with your next overseas flight, why not fight jet lag on home ground. Add Repêchage's bright green, pure Brittany seaweed to your bath, soak for ten minutes and land in better shape. Repêchage Energising Seaweed Bath costs from £49.95.

pool, not for swimming but for aquagym classes. These sea-water exercise classes aim to slim and tone hips, thighs and legs. Each class lasts half an hour, led by an instructor. You can book into Villa Thalgo for a half-day of seaweed and mineral-rich treatments, costing 980 francs, or for a full day,

You lie in a tank while alternating jets of warm and cool sea water massage your body. A mist of seaweed wafts over you throughout. This Vita Cura Treatment aims to oxygenate your blood by stimulating your circulation.

Los Angeles

Aida Thibiant European Day Spa in Beverly Hills is the one to take your body and soul to. Its tree-lined meditation pool and cloud-painted ceilings will make you forget the smog outside as well as in your head.

Madame Thibiant's Aroma Hydromassage Shower, used in all body treatments, is patented. Her skin-care line is both serious, with pharmaceutical-grade glycolic acid for face peels, and tempting. Try her items exotically scented with Tahitian manoi oil. She believes skin should be treated like a precious piece of artwork. Should you want to splash out to improve yours, book into individual treatments or Madame Thibiant's full monty: the seven-hour Ultimate Spa Sanctuary Day ($450). A friend who knows says it's worth it.

Paris

Villa Thalgo day spa is in the heart of Paris, and is dedicated to giving you the best thalassotherapy treatments in an urban setting, using Thalgo products. There is a small sea-water

from 1,700 francs. If you can't get to the sea – and even if you can – try this Parisian delight.

Sydney

The Relaxation Centre in the Hotel Capital is refreshingly rigorous. This is hydrotherapy at its concentrated best. The relaxation comes later. A morning spent here will wake you up without fail: a needle-sharp hose-down, exfoliation, deep tissue massage, scalp therapy, ice-cold cucumber facial, further exfoliation and ten minutes with the Korean masseur or masseuse walking on your back while more water washes away the toxins. I've had this walking-tour massage elsewhere, and alarming as it first seems when the therapist by your side suddenly steps on to your back, it is a form of manipulation that really does work wonders. The Relaxation Centre has separate but equal spas for men and women. Both versions are meant to be equally invigorating. There is a private sleeping room for a nap before the Korean lunch which is included in the price of Aus$60.

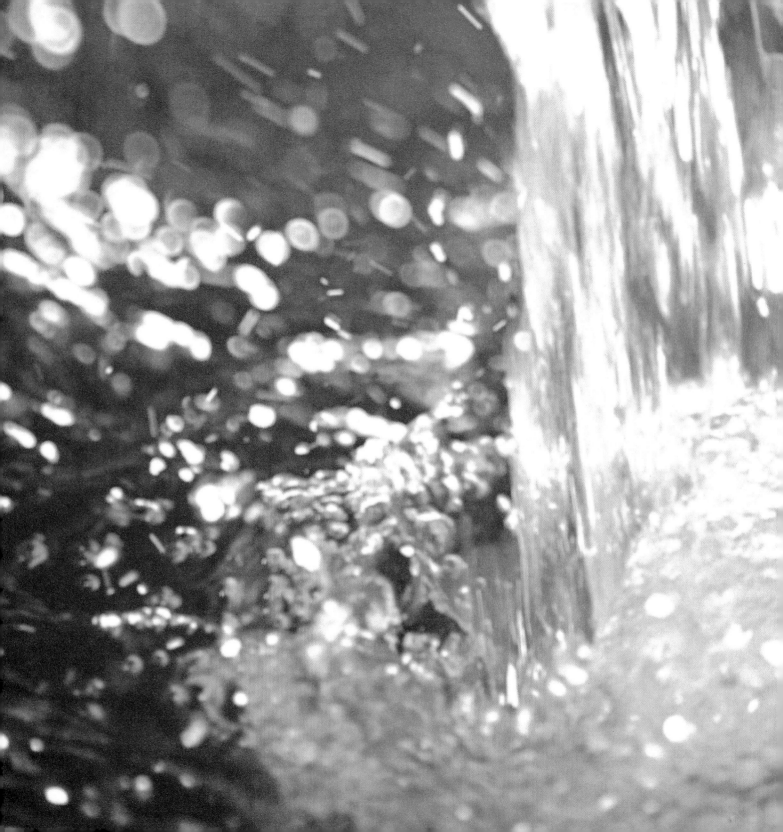

WORLD-CLASS RESIDENTIAL SPAS THAT WILL WATER BODY and SOUL

If you can afford the time and money to go away for a week to a spa, do it. It is a completely worthwhile, rejuvenating experience. Where you go depends on where you are now, geographically, mentally and physically.

Some spas are all inclusive such as Inchydoney in Ireland (see Directory on pages 152–4). This means that treatments are included with your hotel stay. In the case of Inchydoney, Forest Mere in Hampshire and many other spas, where your stay and the treatment centre are all under one roof. Other spas work differently. In Europe, you can often stay somewhere near the treatment institute and simply pay for the treatments either by the day or by the week. This can be cheaper, although it is always more relaxing to be able to walk directly from your hotel room to a treatment room and back again without having to change, get into a car and so on.

If you decide not to use an agent to book your spa, make sure you understand the type of place it is, and what it costs before taking the plunge. Among the hundreds of new and traditional residential spas throughout the world there is at least one just right for you. Establish your needs and your budget. Then think which country you would like to visit – after all, it's a holiday! Consult the consultants, the websites, the books (see page 154) and, of course, ask your friends. Meanwhile, here is a taster to set your spa-minded travel thoughts in motion. Each spa is situated either at a natural spring or on a beach and represents a unique experience. Decide which type whets your appetite: civilised, exotic, invigorating or spiritual.

Domaine du Royal Club Evian

Evian is synonymous with excellent mineral water. Here is an ideal place to drink it while watering body and soul. Luxury never comes cheap and this is no exception. The Hotel Royal is casual/smart (men are required to wear a jacket at dinner) and combines old-fashioned comfort and true style with hi-tech efficiency. You can ask for any level of fitness and beauty regime you want, from gentle to rigorous. All treatments take place at the Institut Mieux-Vivre within the hotel. These include a wide variety of expertly delivered hydrotherapy methods and massage. There is a six day package with three treatments a day for £330. This price stays the same no matter what season you choose. The price of your room in the Hotel Royal is separate from the treatment package and varies according to season and type of accommodation. A single room starts at £73 per person per night.

This is a luxurious European spa resort which will pamper and feed you in more ways than one. The food is Michelin-starred in La Toque Royale restaurant, so if weight loss is your goal, this might not be the perfect spa...

The town of Evian is very relaxing. You can see Lausanne across Lake Geneva and go there in minutes by motorboat. The city of Geneva, just forty minutes up the road, guarantees world-class shopping, – providing yet another kind of therapy! Alone or with a companion, a week here would relax you in a most civilised way.

Chiva-Som International Health Resort

A limo service from Bangkok airport brings you to Chiva-Som, currently considered the ultimate in spa experiences. You will find elegant teak pavilions alongside a beach, with main-building suites overlooking one of two swimming pools.

Wander in and out of the open-air marble rooms decorated with antique Thai friezes, relax to the soothing sounds of rustling palms, sit and gaze into reflecting pools, or get personal instruction in yoga and t'ai chi in an outside pavilion.

There is a multi-level steam room, a flotation room, a hydrotherapy suite, fifteen treatment rooms and a state-of-the-art gym. The staff-to-guest ratio is four to one, so serious pampering is available all day and there is no need for a structured programme. You are left to your own devices and can choose whichever treatments you need. The Thai massage seems reason enough to go there. Apparently the masseuses train with Thai monks for six years.

The approach is holistic, relaxed and informal. You can, if you like, take an energetic walk to nearby waterfalls and beyond in the conservation areas. The surroundings are lush and green, and the food is green as well – all-organic ingredients, presented in a simple, sophisticated East-West fusion style by Australian-born chef Andrew Jacka.

They promise you will lose weight, and that all you will take home is a better body, a more relaxed mind and Jacka's new cookbook to keep you on track. The cost is from £1,200 a week including all food and treatments.

Thalassa Quiberon, Brittany, France

This thalassotherapy centre at the tip of southern Brittany on the Quiberon Peninsula is a classic example of one of ten Thalassa Institutes run by Thalassa International. Each institute in this group is located either by the sea 'or where the purity of the water is excellent'. The other nine are at Le Touquet, Dinard, Carnac, Les Sables-D'Olonne, Oléron, Biarritz, Port-Camargue, Hyères and Porticcio.

Thalassotherapy is carried out under medical supervision with a curative and preventative goal, and to make the most of the treatments you should stay at least six days. But you can choose from a range of shorter, à la carte programmes. Quiberon and several of the other venues are sufficiently convenient to travel to from the UK. For example, if you opt for Quiberon, you can fly from London to Dinard in two hours from £60 return with Ryan Air. (By train from Paris to nearby Auray takes three and a half hours.) A weekend of thalassotherapy at Quiberon is possible, in other words.

The institute is where your treatments take place. You have a choice of three hotels close by: Sofitel Thalassa and Sofitel Dietetique are directly opposite the Thalassa Institute. They offer four-star luxury and face the sea. At the Sofitel Dietetique all meals are individually planned under the supervision of staff dieticians, following a personalised prescription established by nutritional specialists. This is France, so it will not be bread and water! The brochure describes it as 'a marriage of dietetics and gastronomy which leaves the guest without hunger or frustration'. The two-star Hotel Ibis Thalassa is 150 m from the Institute, has an indoor heated pool and Turkish bath and is in a garden setting.

When you arrive at the Thalassa Institute, you will be examined by a qualified medical team. A personal programme will be devised, based on four treatments a day. The Slimming Course, for example, includes whirlpool baths; multijet baths in wrack seaweed-enriched sea water which is noted for its ability to detox; jet showers; underwater sea water showers to firm up the tissues; massages; dynamic swimming treatment, which involves exercising in water; and seaweed packs. You will also have a daily cryothermal (cold/hot) treatment to reduce cellulite. They use Thalocéan products exclusively and you can buy them only at the institute. There is unlimited access to fitness classes, both in and out of the specially equipped pool. There is even a one-hour lesson in low-calorie cookery each day. This particular programme is on a full-board basis only, for a minimum of six days, although nine days is recommended for best results. There is also a men's fitness course which includes thalassotherapy treatment sessions and invigorating swimming sessions, combined with daily sporting activities such as jogging, gymnastics, muscle toning and cardiotraining.

Britanny is ideal for sailing, walking, cycling and horse riding. Even a brisk walk along the beach each day, breathing in the invigorating sea air, is excellent exercise and good for your soul. The expanse of ocean and beach contributes in no

There thermal waters rise from the earth. This is the oldest health spa in North America. ('Ojo' means 'eye'; 'caliente' means 'hot'. Whether 'hot eye' refers to the sun or to the thermal waters, is not clear. The Tewa Indians have visited these springs since the thirteenth century.

The no-frills approach at this spa aims to help you achieve a healthier mind and body in an austerely beautiful setting. If you have never stayed in the desert, this could be the place to begin. The heat itself will relax you and the absence of distraction helps you to look inward, at the same time encouraging you to pay closer attention to nature. A desert landscape is never still if you learn how to listen and look.

You will be drinking from the Lithia spring pump. The

Each institute in this group is located either by the sea 'or where the purity of the water is excellent'

small part to the total beneficial effect of thalassotherapy.

The cost varies according to your hotel, type of room, length of stay, package of treatments and season. The combinations are endless! Here are two examples: Hotel Sofitel Thalassa at Quiberon begins at £684 per person for six nights based on two people sharing a double room on a half-board basis; Thalassa Biarritz offers a weekend break at Hotel Regina et du Golf from £185 per person based on two people sharing a double room and includes two nights with bed and breakfast, two meals for two (lunch or dinner) and three treatments each day.

Ojo Caliente Mineral Springs Resort

In New Mexico, where water has always been precious, equidistant from Santa Fe and Taos, you will find Ojo Caliente.

water is said to lessen depression. Included in the price of your room is access to all seven natural thermal pools, which range in temperature from 49°C (120°F) for the hottest, down to 45°C (113°F). The coolest is the arsenic pool, in fact not poisonous as you would expect, but said to benefit arthritis, rheumatism and stomach ulcers. Along with this is access to a hot tub (again arsenic) and a milagro (meaning 'miracle' in Spanish) wrap treatment: a 'dry wrap' in a cotton, then wool blanket, following the thermal water treatment, to intensify perspiration and help you detox. All other treatments are extra and bookable by the day or as a package. The Ultimate Ojo package includes seven treatments in one day. Prices start at £45 per person per night in the hotel or £60 in a cottage. Mexican, vegetarian and Italian food is served in the spa's restaurant. You will feed body and soul well here.

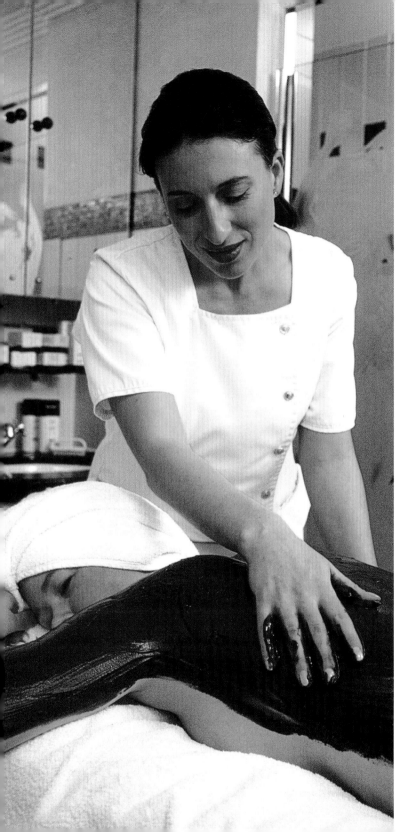

ERNA LOW'S SPA TREATMENT GLOSSARY

Acupuncture	An ancient form of Chinese medicine using the meridian points of the body to channel energy, normally involving the insertion of needles into these points.
Affusion showers	Manual massage carried out under a shower of small sea-water jets: relaxing and soothing.
Algae wraps	Relaxing treatment involving covering the body in various oils and gels and then wrapping in a sheet steamed in algae. Toxins and excess fluids are thus perspired from the body.
Algotherapy	The therapeutic use of algae, usually in conjunction with other marine products. Used to soothe and relax and for anti-inflammatory purposes.
Aquaexercise	Gentle gymnastics in the water, sometimes using underwater jets to increase resistance and tone up the muscles.
Aromatherapy	A pressure-point massage using essential oils with therapeutic properties.
Bubbling baths	Natural sea water enriched with marine mud or seaweeds, or natural thermal waters, which bubble to massage and relax.
Electrotherapy	Therapy involving the use of high-current energy in the form of radio waves to treat internal tissues.
Fango packs	Application of mud mixed with spa water, heated and covered with a plastic sheet to retain the warmth. Recommended for arthritis and rheumatism.
Foaming baths	See Bubbling baths.
G5 massage	A deep, gyratory mechanical massage, good for toning and relaxation.
Hammam	See Steam baths.

Hydromassage	Therapeutic massage involving use of warm water.
Hydrotherapy	Therapeutic treatment involving water.
Inhalation therapy	Inhalation of vapours from sea or thermal waters. Used to help breathing problems and for relaxation.
Jet showers	Massage from a distance using a jet of water held by a supervisor, usually to stimulate circulation.
Lymph drainage	Treatment to help increase the flow of lymphatic fluid carrying waste and toxins from the body. May be in the form of massage, brushing or pressurised leg wraps.
Massage	Body treatment which involves stroking, kneading and pummelling with scented oils. Good for relaxation and muscle relief.
Pressure point therapy	Elimination of toxins by mechanical lymphatic drainage. The process is preceded by a circulatory massage and followed by a cold fango wrap.
Rasul bath	Bath containing three different types of mud – volcanic, peat and Dead Sea – which you massage into your body. Good for cleansing and relaxation.
Reflexology	Relaxing treatment concentrating on massage and applying pressure to different areas of the feet: these connect via energy channels to every organ of the body. Used as a remedial and preventative treatment.
Reiki	Hands-on energy therapy from Japan. Used to help restore balance and harmony to body and mind.
Sauna	A dry heat treatment to help cleanse the body and relax the muscles, usually followed by a cold plunge or shower.
Scottish shower	Jet shower using alternating hot and cold water.
Seamud	Similar to Fango packs but using marine mud and sea water.
Shiatsu massage	A light finger-pressure oriental massage concentrating on the meridian points in the body to channel energy. Watsu is the underwater version of this.
Steam bath	Wet heat treatment using steam to increase perspiration and to aid removal of body toxins.
Submarine showers	Underwater jets to massage and tone the muscles.
T'ai chi	An ancient oriental system of exercise which incorporates self-control and harnesses energy to promote balance, health, harmony and peace. Also used in self-defence.
Thalassotherapy	Therapeutic use of seawater, sea muds, seaweeds and sand with preventative or curative aims in mind.
Thermal baths	Therapeutic use of thermal waters which are rich in salts, bromide, iodine and gases.
Turkish bath	Series of hot and humid steam rooms, each of which increases in heat. You spend several minutes in each room and finish with a tepid or cool shower.
Underwater massage	Massage using high-pressure water jets within a warm-water bath.
Yoga	Indian exercise system to train the mind and body, usually using posture and breathing exercises.

Many thanks to spa specialist Erna Low for permission to reprint this glossary.

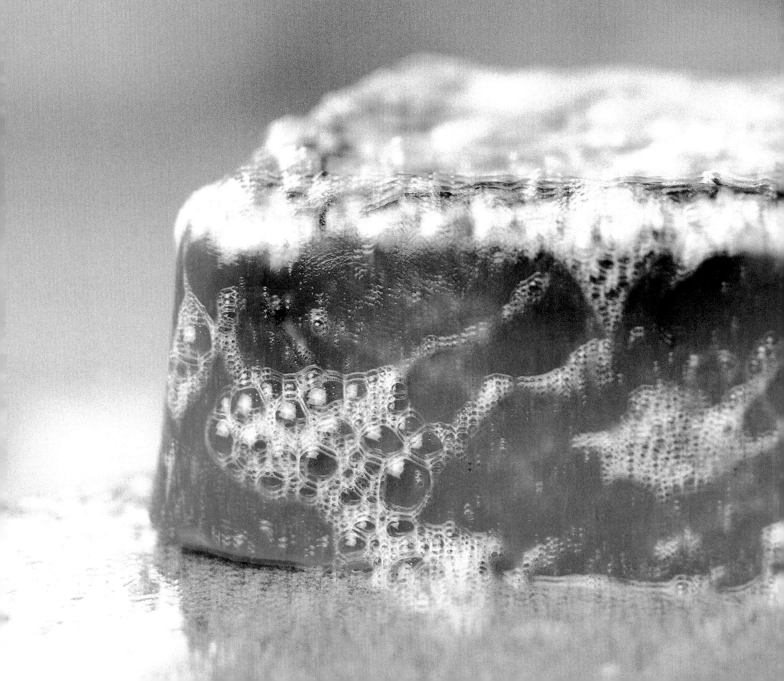

WHATEVER YOUR BEAUTY ROUTINE, JUST ADD

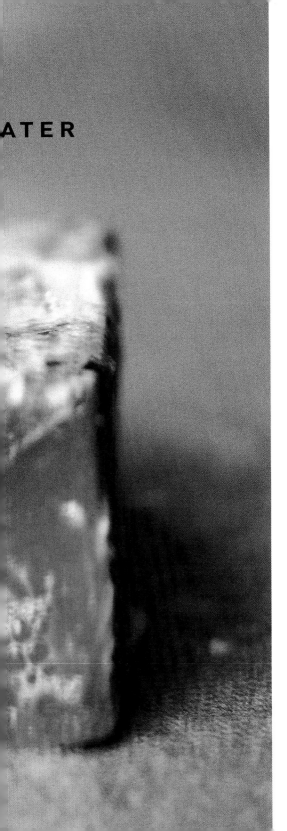

ATER

'Narcissus, wearied with hunting in the heat of the day, lay down here: for he was attracted by the beauty of the place, and by the spring. While he sought to quench his thirst, another thirst grew in him, and as he drank, he was enchanted by the beautiful reflection that he saw.'

METAMORPHOSES
OVID. BOOK III

When supermodel Amber Valletta discussed her beauty routine in *Zest* magazine, water featured prominently. Amber washes her face 'with water and a bar of mild soap'. Constant jet travel dries out her already-dry skin so she sleeps en route as much as possible, moisturises throughout the flight 'and, yes, I really do drink lots of water'. And to revive her skin the morning after? 'I swear by cold water. Splashing it over my face for about two to three minutes gives my circulation a jolt and puts the colour back into my complexion.'

The pure therapy of water isn't reserved for supermodels. Water, if you use it inside and out, can improve your skin's texture and condition with such little effort and expense that it would be folly not to make it integral to your beauty routine. Water goes a long way towards preventing premature dry skin and wrinkles. I've noticed a definite improvement in my own skin since drinking 2 litres (3½ pints) a day. In this section you'll learn how water can help your skin from the inside and out:

- First, why you should drink water to keep your skin looking good.

- Second, how to brush up your morning shower or bath routine to stimulate your lymphatic system and give your skin more than just a glow.

- Third, why you should take a look at new and classic therapeutic skin-care lines based on the unique benefits of sea and fresh water. Learn why Dr Erno Laszlo became world-famous for his 'thirty splashes' and set the stage for skin-care routine as we know it. Why Avène preparations, made for sensitive skin with the waters from the Avène spa, have for years been recommended by dermatologists throughout Europe.

(These are now available in Britain.) And for seaweed-based skin care, dip into the briny with Algascience, Repêchage, Thalgo and Thalocéan.

- Finally, a New Yorker's relaxing, efficient way to water your body from head to toe in just twenty minutes.

DRINK TO BETTER SKIN

While there is always debate among skin specialists and beauty gurus about soap and water versus creams for cleansing, there is total agreement that drinking water is essential for maintaining and improving your skin's clarity, texture and condition. Why is drinking water crucial? New York City dermatologist Debra Jaliman joins the chorus of nutritionists, doctors and skin specialists when she points out that only by drinking enough water (your daily 2 litres) will your skin receive its fair share. The body's major internal organs will always have first call on your body's water supply, so if you skimp, your skin will have to make do with what's left.

Your body needs water on a daily basis to eliminate wastes and toxins. It's because water is such an amazing solvent that your body can excrete chemicals and nitrogenous wastes easily in soluble form without allowing your kidneys to become overloaded. By drinking enough water you are also enabling your skin to retain enough moisture for itself.

Every advertisement for moisturisers makes claims about hydrating and rehydrating your skin. Creams can help your skin retain moisture, but if there is insufficient moisture within your skin's inner layer (called the dermis) to begin with, you will be wasting your money on expensive creams. Drinking enough water each day will help keep fine lines and wrinkles at bay because the reserves of water in the dermis will plump out those line and wrinkles, making them less visible. As you grow older, your skin becomes drier – fight back with water! Whatever your age, whether or not you have a tendency to dry skin, make extra sure that you drink your daily 2 litres.

A lack of water will deplete your skin's reserves and make it look lifeless. But just as it is hard to grasp the long-term effects of smoking on your lungs, which you cannot see, it is equally difficult to understand that your skin is becoming dehydrated and that this is gradually affecting its texture and condition. Take the example of air travel. When you fly, the cabin air is low on oxygen as well as very dry, and this causes short-term dehydration – usually you see and feel it. That's why you should drink lots of water during a flight and avoid spirits and coffee.

Long-term dehydration is like subjecting your skin to a never-ending plane journey. Because unless you work outdoors and have neither central heating nor air-conditioning, you probably spend 90 per cent of each twenty-four-hour day, on average, within a public or private space in which the climate is artificially controlled: your home, car, office, store, shopping centre, cinema, museum and so on. Ultimately this is a very drying (and trying)

situation for your skin – like being on a plane forever! Add a dollop of pollution during your brief sortie into the great outdoors, and you get the picture. If you smoke, your skin suffers even more, because of oxygen depletion. And crash diets don't help either. All this is without overdoing the suntan on holiday.

When it comes to health and beauty, prevention is easier, cheaper and less painful than cure. Dr Gerald Imber, a top New York cosmetic surgeon who has performed thousands of face lifts, is nonetheless all for prevention. He has written a book called *The Youth Corridor* in which he describes this 'youth corridor' as a twenty-five-year period, between the ages of thirty-five and sixty, during which you can remain 'virtually unchanged' if you follow the route of prevention. Why not do everything you can to prevent skin damage and premature ageing, and maintain your skin's health and beauty? Don't crash diet, don't smoke, drink water and read his book.

In it Dr Imber also comes out against running as exercise because 'the rising and pounding lifts and pulls the facial skin away from the underlying muscles and bones': one more reason to learn to swim better? He asks you to 'think of your skin like a pair of tights. After exposure to the elements, multiple washings and thousands of bends and folds, the tights begin to sag. This is strong motivation to take a holistic approach to skin care, starting now. Water alone will not solve the skin-assaulting factors of the twenty-first-century way of life. However, if you can stay well hydrated on the inside, you are doing a lot towards helping your skin maintain its clarity and tone.

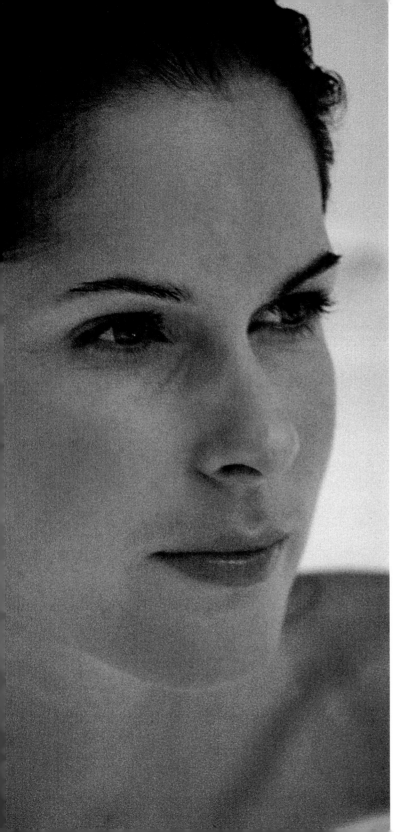

BEGIN YOUR DAY BY BRUSHING YOUR SKIN

Who needs one more thing to do in the morning? But this is so easy, so helpful to your skin's overall condition, and makes you feel so good, that it will soon seem as necessary as brushing your teeth. You always have time for that, don't you? Your skin is the largest organ of your body, but probably your face gets all your attention because it's on view all the time. So you may be neglecting 95 per cent of your skin. In winter this is easily done. Unless you live in the tropics, you are covered in layers of clothes most of the year, which is why swimming all year round or taking a winter break to a hot country is a good idea. It spurs you into taking better care of your body because the thought of getting into a swimsuit tends to concentrate your mind on the shape you are in. Importantly, keeping up an exercise routine throughout the year prevents you from crash dieting every spring.

Daily brushing is important for two reasons: it exfoliates your skin, allowing the pores to eliminate the toxins carried through your circulatory system; and it stimulates your lymphatic system, a fairly static system of fluid which needs your help in order to keep it moving. The main function of the lymphatic system is to drain and eliminate waste and toxins, but unlike your arterial circulatory system, which has your heart to pump the blood around the body, there is no such 'motor' for the lymphatic fluid – that's why it needs help. Lymphatic fluid carries waste material from your cells via lymph vessels which enter your lymph nodes. (You are probably most aware of lymph nodes when you have an infection or sore throat.) Lymph nodes process, or filter, this fluid. Once it is filtered, the cleansed lymphatic fluid leaves the nodes, eventually rejoining the bloodstream at the base of your neck. Lymph nodes are mainly concentrated in your

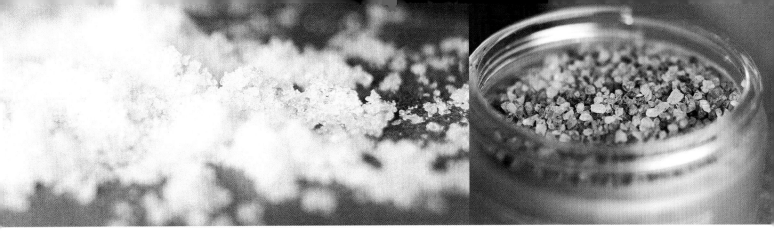

neck, armpits, chest, abdomen and groin, and because they are a key cleansing mechanism for your body, they have an important role in maintaining a strong immune system.

Exercise is vital in order to keep your lymphatic system moving. A healthy diet, massage and skin brushing are the other key ways to help yourself. Try to do all four, especially if you have pockets of cellulite, which is simply fat that gets trapped if your lymphatic drainage is poor. For massage I recommend the Clarins Paris Method, a salon treatment specifically devised for lymph drainage. Meanwhile, treat yourself in your home spa each day with this simple method of skin (or body) brushing.

You will need a good, fairly stiff, natural-bristle brush. The principle is to brush towards your heart, because the valves of the lymphatic nodes go that way.

Starting from your feet, brush slowly but vigorously up your calves and thighs in long, firm strokes, paying special attention to areas where cellulite accumulates; then up along your abdomen and as well as you can up along your buttocks. Next, brush down your back and shoulders and along each arm, especially if the backs of your arms have begun to get flabby, and onwards to the tips of your fingers. Now, starting at your collarbone, brush down towards your heart. That is all there is to it.

Do this *before* your bath or shower, on dry skin, so that the dead skin cells, which you will be loosening up, are washed away. Take care if you have broken skin anywhere – obviously avoid those areas – or if your skin is ultra-sensitive. The exfoliating effect of brushing helps your skin renew itself. If you have a dull, end-of-season tan, it will help your skin look fresh.

(For a 21-day natural detox plan, and information on foods which can help keep the lymphatic system clear, read Helene Silver's helpful book *Rejuvenate*, and her chapter 'Lymph: The Hidden Ocean Within'.)

USE THERAPEUTIC SKIN-CARE PREPARATIONS INSPIRED BY WATER
Erno Laszlo

Dr Erno Laszlo became famous for asking women to splash their faces with 'dirty' water. He was the first to recognise the extraordinary benefits of water and the originator of the concept that water, not oil, naturally replenishes the skin. Through his dermatological research, he realised that water was vital in order to maintain hydration levels in your skin and that it can prevent premature ageing. He devised a system which personalised a skin-care 'ritual' for every skin type. According to the Laszlo company, this approach is the inspiration for most of today's skin care and make-up treatment lines, including Clinique.

Whatever your skin type, Laszlo's signature technique is water – thirty splashes in all. Throw away your face flannel. Use his soap directly on your face. Then, for the first twenty treatment splashes, you use comfortably hot or warm water depending on your individual skin type. These are meant to maximise the effect of the beneficial properties of the Erno Laszlo skin-care products. These 'treatment' splashes are done with the plug in the sink, so you are splashing your face with soapy ('dirty') water. Why? Dirt and lather bonds with oil, so as you splash again and again from the basin of now-soapy water, this rich emulsion is more effective at picking up the dirt on your skin than plain water, and results in cleaner, fresher skin.

This is followed by ten splashes of fresh running water to gently remove final impurities and to hydrate your skin.

mysterious sanctuary in which women felt transformed by the doctor's advice, personal prescriptive routines and overall methods. The institute's elegant treatment rooms were decorated in jet black with touches of cream – like his product labels – because Laszlo felt black was 'the most restful colour'. The assistants matched the interior, wore black dresses and spoke in hushed tones – in English with strong Hungarian accents. (The Duchess of Windsor called the Institute 'the house of silence'!) Laszlo demanded of each client that she (or sometimes he) tell the utter truth about how she lived her life – diet, smoking, exercise, sex – before he could treat her skin. He was the first to understand that your skin changes according to diet, emotions, exercise, or lack of it, as well as from season to season, and that you have to treat it accordingly. The most common and unexpected question the doctor asked was: 'When was the last time you washed your face?' Many had never used soap

'Water, with the right kind of soap is the basis of every beauty routine. If it weren't already invented, I would have had to invent it myself!'

Laszlo became a legendary figure in the world of skin care who rose to cult status even before he gained the utter devotion of celebrities like Marilyn Monroe, Greta Garbo, Audrey Hepburn and Jackie Onassis. Generations later, the client list is still star-studded and includes Barbra Streisand, Madonna, Sting – the names go on and on.

Laszlo studied under Professor Max Joseph, considered to be the father of modern dermatology. Laszlo opened his Institute of Cosmetology in Budapest in 1927 and then a replica of it in New York City in 1939. Each was an elegant,

and water. 'Let me tell you, dear lady,' Laszlo would begin, 'if water were uncommon, it would be worth its weight in gold. You would treasure it in crystal bottles and speak of its magical powers with bated breath. Water, with the right kind of soap is the basis of every beauty routine. If it weren't already invented, I would have had to invent it myself!' He believed in water so completely that none of his clients could continue with him unless they learned to wash their faces in the proper way. Until then, he said, 'you cannot know the healing powers of water'.

Here are the eight key benefits of water according to Laszlo:

- Exfoliates skin cells.
- Accelerates cellular renewal
- Flushes out damaging toxins
- Plumps and softens skin
- Enhances the absorption of moisturisers
- Exercises and strengthens capillaries
- Deeply and thoroughly cleanses skin
- Stimulates collagen production

Diana Jewell, in her informative and entertaining biography, *The Angel of Beauty* (sadly not for sale as it was a limited edition publication) explains that Laszlo 'knew that the wealthiest of ancient Eastern civilisations had the luxury of water; the peasants did not. Clean, scrupulous skin was more than a sign of great riches, it was the result of the restorative benefits of water on the skin. Yet even the most privileged women in America simply did not wash their faces; it was not the fashion. And their skin was suffering because of it.'

Water is the least expensive element of the Laszlo story. His 'preparations' – never products – are very pricey, but they are extraordinarily gentle and effective. (The eye make-up remover is relatively affordable at £16. The Intensive Firming Complex is a steep £65.) There are wonderful soaps to choose from. Or you could do the thirty-splash soap-and-water technique with your own bar. And while you are counting splashes, consider this: Laszlo splashed his own face with water at least ninety times a day.

Avène

The Avène Thermal Spa in the south-west of France near Montpellier has been visited since the 1700s, and in 1975 the Pierre Fabre Laboratories carried out a systematic study of the waters. Their research showed that the particular composition of these spa waters, low in minerals and high in silica – making them very soft – is therapeutic for a wide range of skin problems, including eczema, psoriasis, and irritable, itchy skin. Skin sensitivity can be caused by many different factors at different times of your life: cold weather, a new detergent, a fragrance, cosmetic or preservative that suddenly triggers an allergic reaction.

The Avène Spa treats around 1500 people a year, and reports a 90 per cent success rate with the redness, itching and discomfort disappearing. If you are French, you can go to the spa on recommendation from your doctor and be treated free. If you are not French, the spa treatment is very reasonably priced, costing from £200 for three weeks. Many families turn their visit into a holiday and camp nearby. This is not a pampering spa: you will need a doctor's prescription. However, it is in a very beautiful spot, with the River Orb flowing through the lovely village. Because so many children suffer from eczema, the summer holiday period is a very busy time. Plan ahead.

Pierre Fabre, a pharmacist by profession, launched the Avène skin-care range which became number one in France, is recommended by dermatologists throughout Europe and is now available in Britain. All the products are made at the spa. There is an Eau Thermale (£5) which would refresh anyone's skin – a fine mist spray with all the anti-irritating properties of the soft spa water.

The best in seaweed-based treatments

Seaweed is the new buzzword in beauty treatments. The question to ask is not why, but why now? Excellent plant

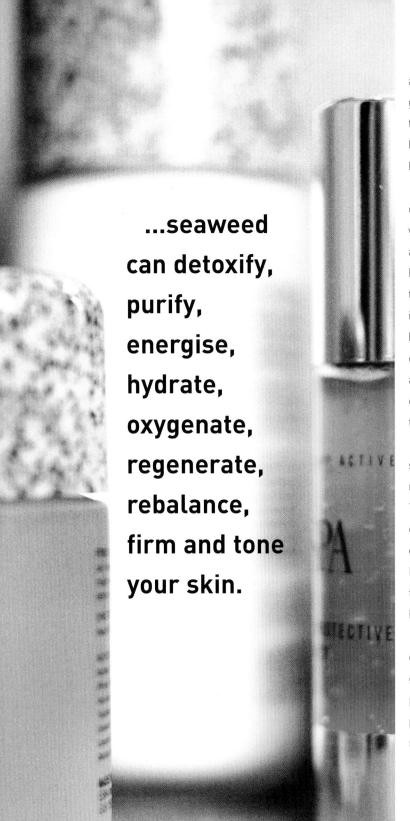

...seaweed can detoxify, purify, energise, hydrate, oxygenate, regenerate, rebalance, firm and tone your skin.

and herbal-based preparations such as Clarins have been going strong for decades. It seems simply that now seaweed's time has come. Once again, French companies are taking the lead, as well as an American one with a French name, Repêchage.

Seaweed is a concentration of sea water. When it is crushed and micronised properly, all the elements of sea water are concentrated 'to between 5,000 and 50,000 times according to a leading expert in this field, Dr Christine Bodeau-Bellion. What are these elements? As explained in the section on thalassotherapy (sea-water therapy), sea water is more than just salty water. It is composed of highly beneficial mineral salts including magnesium, potassium and calcium, amino acids, vitamins A, B1, B2, B12, C, D, E and K, and trace elements including iron, manganese, boron, copper, aluminium, cobalt and zinc. An impressive list, but do they make you look better?

Lydia Sarfati, the founder of Repêchage, believes that seaweed can detoxify, purify, energise, hydrate, oxygenate, regenerate, rebalance, firm and tone your skin. She explains: 'Seaweed is simply a concentration of sea water that is capable of providing, above any other source, all of the elements needed for the proliferation of healthy skin cells. Repêchage's Four-Layer Facial is well worth an hour of your time. It costs between £30 and £60 depending on where you have it done.

You will find Thalgo or Thalocéan preparations used exclusively at most top thalassotherapy spas. Both are French companies offering quality seaweed and marine-algae based products which are excellent for your skin. To achieve the promised benefits, look for the highest concentration of marine algae: for example, the Thalgo bath concentrate is

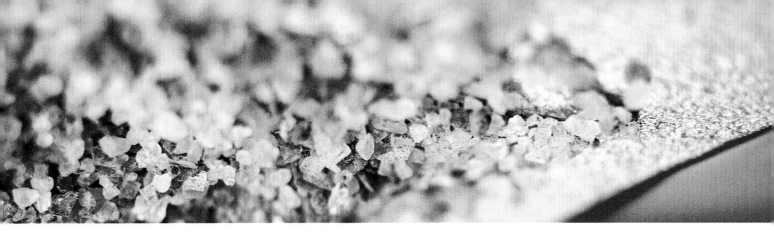

labelled: '100 per cent pure natural micronized marine algae'. Otherwise you could be getting only a tiny percentage of seaweed, some blue-green colouring, foam and some scent from a company that is just jumping on the seaweed boat – or flotilla...

Algascience is the very serious French company created by the prominent marine biologist Dr Christine Bodeau-Bellion. She spent her childhood harvesting seaweed on the Brittany coast and now has two science doctorates, one of them in microbiology. 'I see myself more as a research engineer than a chief executive,' she says, and it seems that she is in the frontier of seaweed-based cosmetology. 'Seaweed cells,' she explains, 'have surprising similarities to those of the human skin, giving rise to the idea among researchers that certain molecules taken from seaweed can be as useful to cosmetology as medicine: an active ingredient capable of synthesising collagen could be the base not only of an anti-ageing cream, but also an anti-scarring agent.'

Algascience uses only deep-water seaweed in its range, as opposed to the shoreline variety. One advantage of this is the improved smell, since some shoreline seaweeds – for example, bladderwrack – smell like very low tide. Again, try anything at all from Christine Bodeau-Bellion's dedicated

company. Why not begin with Relaxing Sea Bath Crystals? These turn your bath water a most beautiful shade of blue – and it is the real thing. A very reasonable £6.95 buys you a 450 g (1 lb) jar, which you can refill with from their 1 kg (21/4 lb) pack. Algascience preparations are available throughout Europe and America only in selected stores where trained skin-care specialists can advise you.

New York's famous Bliss Day Spa (see pages 152–4) offers a wide range of marine-based products, including a seaweed face mask that is Mary Ehni's favourite. Mary is a top Manhattan hair-colourist who recommends the following time-saving method of conditioning your hair while relaxing your body, treating your face and refreshing your eyes – simultaneously.

'First, put on your seaweed mask. Choose the suitable conditioner for your hair type, then apply thoroughly from roots to ends, paying special attention to any over-stressed dry areas. Wrap your hair in plastic or place a plastic cap over it. Soak a towel in the hottest water tolerable, wring it out and wrap around your hair (turban-style). Finish off the look with two cucumber slices over the eyes. Great for reducing puffiness, and it really works! (Pond's make a very good cucumber pad if you don't have a fresh cucumber in the fridge.) Then sit back and relax for 15–20 minutes.'

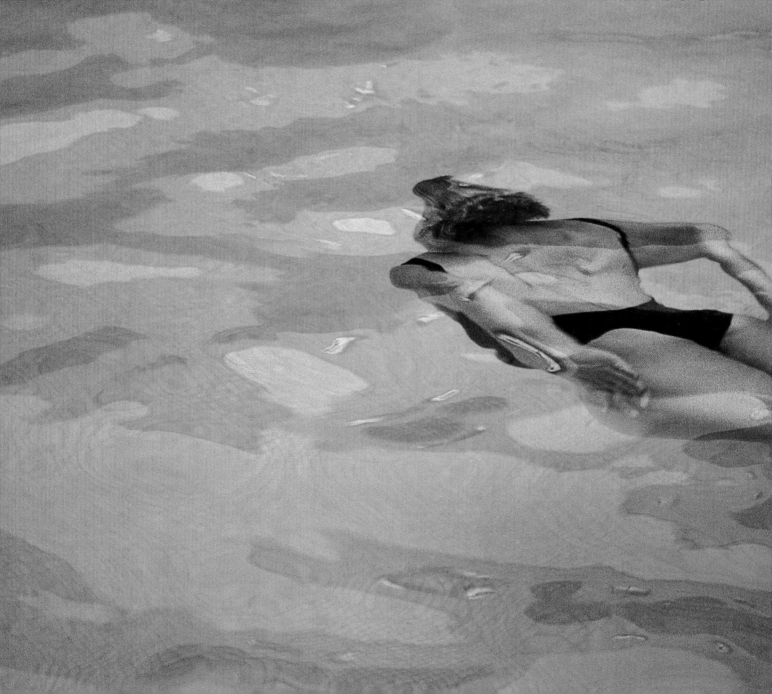

SWIMMING IS BRIMMING WITH BENEFITS

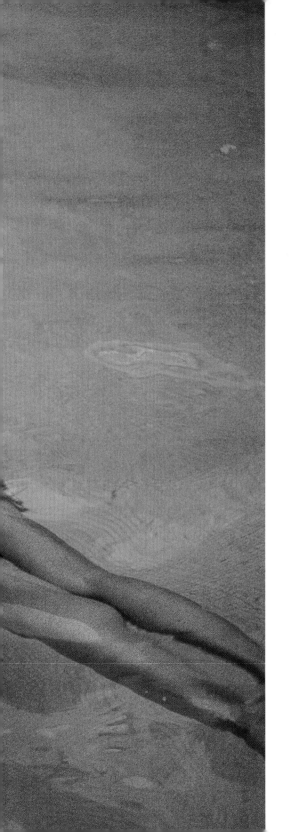

People wish to learn to swim and at the same time to keep one foot on the ground.

MARCEL PROUST
REMEMBRANCE OF THINGS PAST

'Exercising in water is not just physical,' says Jane Katz, 1998 US Masters swimming champion. 'Your mood is enhanced; there's a sense of well-being.' Absolutely – if you're an ace swimmer who glides effortlessly through water, looks lithe in lycra and never clutches the side of the pool gasping for breath, swimming is fantastic exercise and great fun. What about the rest of us?

What if thrashing back and forth in the local pool constitutes your daily swim, the dog paddle remains your best stroke and, worse still, the deep end of a pool, after years of swimming, continues to spell FEAR in capital letters?

Relax. There are new ways to get you into the swim whatever your age and fitness level, from the famous French method which teaches you to breathe correctly by dipping your head in a salad bowl full of water, to the Alexander Technique applied to water. Any method that works for you is worth trying. Also, if you have a new baby, don't wait too long to teach it to swim. Experienced swimming instructors I spoke to believe that five months is the ideal age to begin getting your little one's toes wet.

Swimming is pure joy, pure therapy and terrific exercise. While any kind of exercise is good for you, swimming is probably the best, especially for women. Women's knees and hips are less flexible than men's, so if you are a city-streets jogger, if you play squash or hard sets of tennis, perhaps you should ease up on those sports and add water to your exercise routine in the form of swimming. As a woman, you are much more likely to suffer from acute knee injuries than a man, and knee injuries are known to be linked to the development of osteoarthritis. While swimming, however, you are exercising without putting any load on sensitive joints because your body is supported by the water. No other form of exercise uses so many muscles so fully. Trainers and sports scientists agree that swimming is the ideal way to exercise. Robert McMurray, PhD, professor of sports science at the University of North Carolina at Chapel Hill, sums it up simply. He rates swimming as 'one of the best all-around exercises...it places minimal stress on the joints'.

Swimming has always been part-play, part-exercise, and this is what makes it unique. Of course, since the sea was considered mysterious and dangerous by early coastal peoples, plunging into the waves for fun or exercise was risky and rare. In Britain sea bathing became popular only in the late eighteenth and nineteenth centuries. Why do so many fishermen never learn to swim? Apparently, to know how to swim would only prolong the agony of drowning should their boat capsize in a storm or run aground.

Nonetheless, the ancient Greeks and Romans apparently swam for pleasure as well as exercise – swimming was used to train their warriors (though whether this training took place in rivers or the sea is not clear). In Japan too, as early as the first century BC, swimming competitions were held. However, as the population in various parts of the world began to cluster into larger and larger groups, moving from rural areas where rivers ran clear and pure, to towns and cities, where water became a carrier of disease, swimming gradually began to disappear as a source of pleasure or

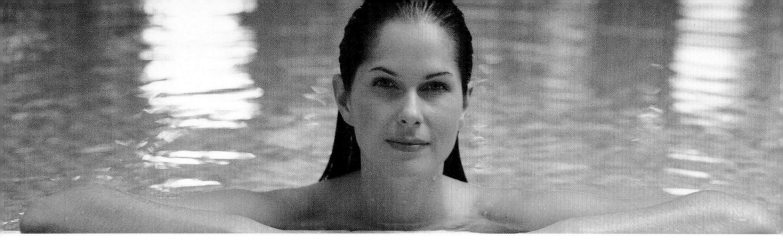

exercise. Certainly in Europe during the Middle Ages, from around the fifth to the fifteenth century, people were far too worried about waterborne fatal diseases, such as the plague and cholera, to immerse themselves in water of any kind. It took several significant scientific discoveries to end these epidemics and to make people feel that it was safe – indeed medicinal – to go for a swim.

The pendulum swung quickly in the other direction. In Britain, for example, people discovered that swimming

as we know it; instead they 'took a dip'. It's an expression we use today which originates from that time.

Meanwhile, the British coastal spas soon developed into the seaside resorts which are still popular, and thanks to the improved roads and the railways, the entrancing, mysterious and distant sea became accessible to all classes, though the surrounding real estate became (and remains) expensive and out of reach. Interestingly the colourful little beach huts strung along the sands at West Whittering (Sussex),

Apparently English summers are getting warmer. Until the change becomes apparent, the word 'bracing' best describes swimming in Britain, from Skegness to the Cornish 'Riviera'!

was indeed so much fun that nude mixed bathing parties became popular in Brighton and Scarborough. When Queen Victoria was told of these wild parties, she was 'not amused' so men and women generally kept on their bathing costumes – and the joy of swimming continued, though no doubt somewhat diminished.

If you have wondered how people could ever stay afloat wearing all those clothes, the answer is that in these early years of sea, lake or river bathing, only a few people 'swam'

Whitstable (Kent) and Camber Sands (Essex), once used as places for the family to perch for the day, are now being bought enthusiastically as simple summer retreats by the British middle classes who have 'been there, done that', and are coming home to their own magnificent coastline, chilly as it is. Apparently English summers are getting warmer.

Until the change becomes apparent, the word 'bracing' best describes swimming in Britain, from Skegness to the Cornish 'Riviera'!

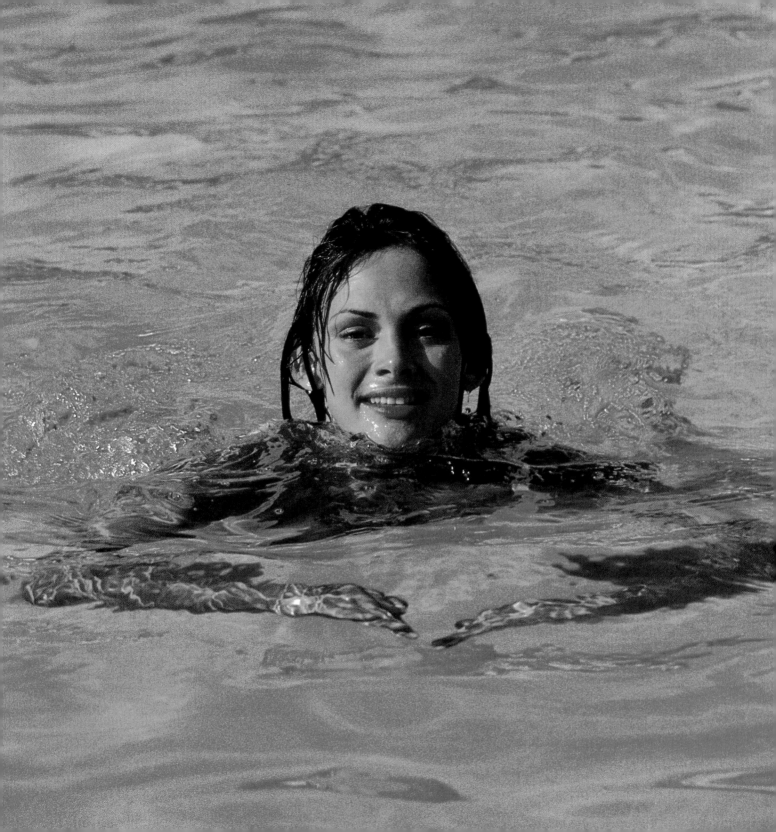

LEARNING TO SWIM

The Motivation

Swimming well can boost your confidence and make you feel truly at one with yourself and with nature. Yes, it's harder to learn as you get older, but there are ways to conquer your fear. Proust was speaking in metaphor, but you do have to learn to let go to become a swimmer. This is precisely why learning to swim is worth the effort, and why swimming truly relaxes you. You have to trust the water; you have to trust its buoyancy. In essence, you have to learn to trust yourself as well as nature.

Women have always excelled at swimming. Women's swimming was brought into the Olympic programme in 1912 in Stockholm, Sweden, and in 1926 the American Gertrude Ederle became the first woman to swim the English Channel. Swimming can be anything from exhilarating to meditative. A half-hour swim each evening can calm and restore you after a stressful working day. A planned routine of swimming can go a long way towards healing you after a physical or psychological illness. Swimming as exercise should be pleasurable, so try not to clock-watch and turn it into another chore.

The mind-and-body-benefits you derive from swimming will depend on how well you swim, but also on where, when, why and how you do it. It's worth planning your swim at a time when your local pool is not crowded – the silence of swimming solo in a pool is incredibly relaxing. As you move through water, your head begins to clear. Let the rhythm of swimming soothe you. It might well become your most creative time of day.

Doing a few lengths in a pool is better than nothing at all, but don't suppose it will burn calories or shape you. It takes around thirty minutes of continuous swimming for your body to recognise it as a workout. (This is true for most types of exercise.) While you are building up your stamina, water aerobics are good fun and excellent exercise. If there is no aerobics class at your local pool, try just walking back and forth at the shallow end (in waist-high water) or holding on to the side of the pool and practising your flutter kick to make up your thirty minutes of continuous exercise.

Exercise continues to make news in terms of maintaining your health and preventing killer diseases such as cancer. According to an eleven-year study of nearly two thousand post-menopausal women in America, those who were the most active – which this study defines as swimming, running or playing tennis at least once a week – were 80 per cent less likely to develop breast cancer. Of these active ways to exercise, swimming is the least stressful on your joints.

If you haven't learned how to swim, make this your year to take the plunge. If you can swim but not very well (and as a result don't really enjoy it), take heart: apparently only 5 per cent per cent of swimmers know how to move and use their limbs and body correctly. It is not easy in a cold country to keep up a swimming routine, especially in winter. Swimming with a friend can help. On cold, rainy nights when the idea of shedding your clothes and jumping into a pool definitely does not beckon, you can encourage each other.

You always feel so much better after a swim. Just as drinking water becomes easier and easier as you do it, until your body longs for its daily 2 litres, your body will soon begin to look forward to its restorative swim. Perhaps a short spell of lessons, more practice in relaxed surroundings, even a video to help you along could make swimming your most enjoyable form of exercise. Swimming well will give you the confidence to enjoy sea and fresh-water sports on your next holiday.

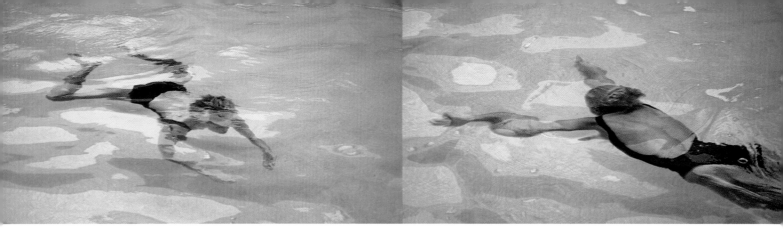

The Method

Five strokes constitute modern-day swimming: breaststroke, crawl (freestyle), backstroke, butterfly and sidestroke.

Breaststroke This is the oldest style of swimming, known since the seventeenth century. It challenges your lower body the most. Lying on your front, the arms are pointed straight ahead then swept backwards in line with the shoulders. Simultaneously the legs are drawn up to the body with knees and toes pointed out, then are thrust back as the elbows draw into the side of the ribs. If you have a lot of tension in your neck and shoulders, it is not advisable to make this your favourite stroke, even if you do it properly so that you exhale underwater. Breaststroke can make things even more tense and difficult for your neck and shoulders because of the position your head is in most of the time: cricked up at an acute angle for length after length of swimming. Your head is heavy and your neck and shoulders will bear the burden of it.

Crawl (freestyle) This is an enviable stroke to know and beautiful to observe. It was developed in the 1870s by the English swimmer John Arthur Trudgen. Proper breathing is critical to this stroke which requires not only practice but also professional lessons in order to learn it well. The flutter kick is important with this stroke to keep your lower body buoyant. (Alternate your legs' up-and-down movement from the hips, not the knees, with relaxed, not stiff, legs.) The arms move, alternately, through the air, the hand turning palm down to catch the water with the elbow bent while the other arm pulls back under the water. The crawl involves two to eight kick strokes per single arm movement. Your head should always be resting in the water; turn it sideways to inhale, then exhale underwater. (You will see how one instructor suggests you practise this stroke in a salad bowl.) The crawl works your upper body most of all.

Backstroke Flip onto your back from the crawl and relax. Again, you use the flutter kick to propel you, with alternate arms lifted and returned to your side to pull your body through the water. I find this stroke immensely relaxing, except in a rough sea when waves wash over your face and you inhale a mouthful of salt water! This stroke was first used in the 1912 Olympic Games by Harry Hebner, an American swimmer. I sometimes do a variation on this stroke to give my upper body extra exercise. I move only my arms, without moving my legs. This gives the upper arms, which tend to hold a lot of fat deposits, an excellent workout.

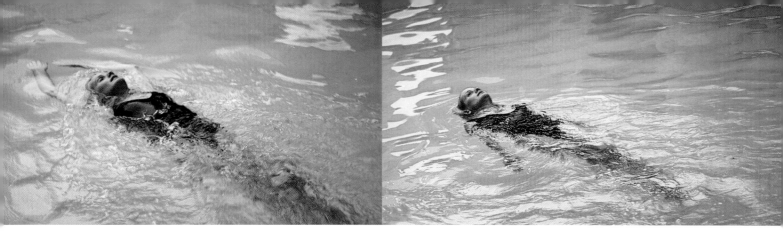

Butterfly A variation of breaststroke, but I think much more difficult unless you swim competitively. This would not be a stroke to concentrate on to enhance your level of fitness or to relax. The leg kick is called the dolphin kick: a definite downward motion of your unseparated feet. Both arms are brought forward together over the water then swept backwards simultaneously under the water. This continuous action is accompanied by an undulating movement of the hips. This stroke was developed in the 1930s by the American swimmer Henry Myers and it was recognised in the 1950s as separate from the breaststroke.

thighs. Try to change sides when you do the sidestroke, whether you are doing laps in a pool or swimming outside (assuming the sea is calm, of course), lying first on one side, then on the other, to exercise your whole body evenly. The sidestroke is particularly good at helping to streamline the muscles in your rib cage.

For weight loss or toning your muscles, you have to build up your endurance. Thirty minutes of continuous swimming burns about 250 calories compared to 148 for cycling and 340 for running – at a pace of ten minutes per 1.6km (1mile). These figures are calculated for a woman weighing 63.5kg (10

Thirty minutes of continuous swimming burns about 250 calories compared to 148 for cycling and 340 for running – at a pace of ten minutes per 1.6km (1mile).

Sidestroke This is my favourite. It's ideal for long-distance swimming as well as for life-saving. It used to be a competition stroke but is now used only in non-competitive swimming. It is utterly relaxing and particularly good if you are swimming in the sea on a rough day – just put your back to the waves. You use a sharpish sideways scissor kick to propel you through the water: great exercise for your hips and

stone/140 lb) doing a thirty-minute workout. Mix your strokes and vary your speed for the best overall exercise. Each stroke flexes, stretches and strengthens different joints and muscles. If you add flippers, your body will have to work harder because you will be slightly higher in the water, and more effort will be required of the muscles on the front of your thighs (quadriceps).

THE SALAD-BOWL METHOD

Leave it to the French to use cooking utensils in the most effective ways. The legendary Pierre Gruneberg has taught his ABC of swimming (aquatic breathing control) in the South of France for fifty summers. His pupils read like a who's who of the Western world, and include famous names from every walk of life: Jean Cocteau, Picasso, Somerset Maugham, French rock star Johnny Hallyday, Elton John, Robin Williams, Ralph Lauren and Charlie Chaplin. As well as in France, Gruneberg now also teaches in Britain and America.

If everyone from Cocteau to Chaplin has learned the salad-bowl way, why not you and me? Gruneberg places great

water, practising your breathing in warm and dry surroundings before you go near the pool. Gruneberg teaches you to breathe out through your nose and mouth while your face is in the bowl of water, humming, or as he calls this part of his technique, *chanter dans l'eau*. So you're singing in the water – what could be more pleasurable! You then lift your head out of the bowl and scrunch up your nose, making a rabbit-like face as you sharply exhale the last bit of air. Practice makes perfect, and you have to repeat these breathing exercises many times before you get them right.

Fear of running out of breath is of course what makes most people erratic and poor swimmers. Gruneberg's method makes you realise how long you can hold your breath once

'At the start, I was like everyone else,' he says. 'But I saw the problems people were having and realised we didn't spend enough time teaching breathing.

importance on learning how to breathe and understands, unlike so many teachers, that fear of water stops people from mastering the correct technique, so he doesn't begin his lessons in the water.

'At the start, I was like everyone else,' he says. 'But I saw the problems people were having and realised we didn't spend enough time teaching breathing. But you can't teach breathing in the water. People freeze. They can't see what they are doing and I can't see. So we do it in a salad bowl. They are warm, they can see and I can see and help them. When they have the breathing, the strokes come more easily.

I see lots of good swimmers, but lots of them are bad breathers.'

You spend your first hour with a half-full salad bowl of

you lose your fear of being underwater in the first place – again, by practising holding your breath while keeping your head in the nice, safe salad bowl. Try it today. You'll feel ridiculous but it will convince you that you could learn to breathe deeply and hold your breath for longer. One minute is not hard to do if you're relaxed, and knowing this gives you enormous confidence. You probably have more stamina than you think. Amazingly, top athlete and free-diver Tanya Streeter can hold her breath for as long as *five minutes*. Free-diving (also called breath-hold diving) involves diving with only the oxygen in your lungs, wearing a wet-suit, snorkel, flippers and mask. Tanya Streeter dives 90m (300 ft) into the ocean and back. So. Dipping your head into that salad bowl is a modest beginning.

THE SHAW METHOD

Steven Shaw and his wife Limor apply the principles of the Alexander Technique to teach you to swim without putting stress on your body, particularly on your neck, back and knees, and to make it an enjoyable experience. Shaw observed that many people 'hold their heads up and out of the water, and the pressure squeezes the vertebrae: invariably, many complain of aches and stiffness'. He also noticed how many people 'power crawl' to reach their self-imposed target.... Not only can poor technique lead to neck, back and shoulder trouble, but such swimmers often do not enjoy what they are doing.'

If any of the above sounds familiar, this might be the method for you. The Alexander Technique is excellent for easing neck and back problems and for making you more aware in general of the way you breathe, stand, sit and move. Shaw became so impressed by the results of the Alexander Technique on himself that he trained as an Alexander instructor – and met his wife in the process. Together they developed a way to teach swimming using the Alexander Technique. The Art of Swimming, their video, starts you off on land to build your confidence and train you to relax before you even get into the water. Relaxing in and especially *under* water is, as with Gruneberg's method, the key to good swimming. How do you do it if you are afraid of dunking your head, running out of breath, getting water in your eyes and so on? Shaw has some practical advice: invest in the best pair of goggles you can get – the most up-to-date ones do not leak. As for your other excuses, they will gradually disappear as you relax (they promise!) and find that you won't sink to the bottom the moment you put your head under water. Your breathing will improve as your swimming does.

Breathing out while swimming with your head under water, according to recent research, says Shaw, is good for relieving stress. So it really is worthwhile to learn to swim without stressing your body: forget that stiff-necked breaststroke forever. Shaw also emphasises that swimming should be playful. The video illustrates that he and his wife practise what they preach. They even include Baudelaire's poetry to inspire you – Limor is a former yoga instructor and so the meditative potential of swimming ranks high on the Shaws' list. (See pages 152–4 for details on the availability of lessons.)

Come the darker days of winter, you may be tempted, as I am, to book a swimming holiday with the Shaws on the Red Sea at Nuweba, about an hour from Eilat. You would stay at the five-star Hilton Hotel on a two-meal-a-day basis and receive four hours of swimming instruction daily. This costs from £779 per person for the week, including all instruction, room, meals and flight. You might get to swim with dolphins!

Dip into these organisations in the UK and USA:
Wherever you live in the world, your local pool probably has a list of instructors who can give you lessons. If you need information on any UK-based adult swimming courses contact: The Amateur Swimming Association on +44 (0) 1509-618 719

To find a water-fitness programme in the USA contact:
YMCA : 1-800-USA-YMCA; Aquatic Exercise Association (tel: 001 941 486 8600; or American Physical Therapy Association (tel: 001 703 684 2782)

EARLY DAYS OF 'TAKING A DIP'

Imagine taking a dip at Brighton in the early days of sea bathing. You wouldn't be going for a swim – not as we know it – you would quite literally be dipped into the sea! At Brighton, there were local people called dippers who would lower you into the sea. If you preferred, a bathing machine could roll you in and out of the surf – these were pulled by men or horses. Clearly, no one (apart from the dippers, haulers and horses) benefited much in way of exercise.

Sea bathing in the eighteenth and nineteenth centuries

MAKE YOURS A WATER BABY

Don't you wish you had learned to swim like a baby dolphin from birth? The dolphin, whale and otter, our mammal cousins, are so comfortable in water. Why not give your baby that gift, so your child becomes as one with nature, able to explore and experience the thrill of wild swimming – in rivers, lakes and the sea – as well as exercising in and enjoying the more mundane pleasures of the local pool.

Rachael, a qualified Australian swimming instructor who specialises in teaching babies to swim, and who is also an

Moreover, when babies are playfully dunked in the water and you see them kicking furiously, they are struggling, not swimming (as in drowning, not waving!).

was more for medicinal purposes than for exercise or fun, although of course lots of people did enjoy themselves. Brighton's rise to fame as a sea spa, crowned by its great pavilion, owed its popularity in great part to the Prince of Wales (Prinny) who was keen on sea bathing. However, it was also greatly helped by two local doctors whose publications promoted the benefits of drinking sea water (in small amounts!) as well as dipping into the briny.

In 1752, Dr Richard Russell published *A Dissertation on the Use of Sea Water*, followed a few years later by Dr John Awsiter's publications. He declared that sea-bathing was beneficial for many diseases, and might even cure infertility. Dr Awsiter advised people not to bathe after a big meal and to take a dip at dawn when both mind and body were in a calm state..

experienced nanny, believes that babies do not know how to swim instinctively from birth, however appealing that notion might be. It is true that they are floating in amniotic fluid before birth, but they are not swimming; neither do they know how to swim when they are born. Moreover, when babies are playfully dunked in the water and you see them kicking furiously, they are struggling, not swimming (as in drowning, not waving!). That adorable little frog-leg kick you might interpret as evidence for an instinctive knowledge of swimming, is actually a reaction to fear. Rachael explains that if you scare a baby by dunking it in the water, it will kick its legs, jut out both its arms to the sides and breathe in. If you then lift the baby out of the water and praise it, this begins to teach it to swim. This is indeed how Rachael was taught to teach infants as young as three months old.

However, after many years of teaching and being a nanny, Rachael feels that five months is the ideal age. She is also convinced that an infant or toddler learns best by imitation and by play. So she does not 'teach' the whole time when she is in the water with her little pupil. And *never* does she force a baby's (or child's) face under the water. This can give them a permanent fear of water. Rachael's technique is to put her own face in the water and to blow bubbles. She supports the infant in front of her, arms beneath the infant's arms, and soon the baby begins to blow bubbles too. This imitation technique builds trust and is fun. Trust is all-important, Rachael says, and it is best if the person teaching your baby is someone whom your baby sees more often than just once a week in a potentially scary situation – like a pool.

All this points to the importance of learning to swim well yourself, so that you could learn to teach your little one or at least to recognise a good teacher when you meet him or her.

The best way forward is to ask at your local pool for instructors who specialise in teaching children and, if you can, go along to observe before you commit your own baby to a series of lessons.

FOLLOW A SWIM WITH STEAM

A steam bath uses intense wet heat to draw the toxins out of your pores and relax your muscles. A sauna, which involves dry heat, is less messy, but steam makes you sweat faster and more profusely (sweating is the point) and your skin never feels as crackly dry as it does during and after a sauna.

Taking a steam bath is a fairly lengthy process – much more than just a dip in and out. It can be quite enervating, so don't be tempted to take one too often. Because you are going to subject your body to intense heat, you should make sure you are in good health, (if you have any heart problem, check with your doctor whether the treatment is safe for you) and always take your time and do it gradually. This is why a typical Arabic *hammam* (the origin of the Turkish steam bath) consisted – and still consists – of a series of rooms, each varying in temperature according to the height and shape of the domed roof and to the room's distance from the source of heat. In early days the heat was provided by a furnace or natural thermal waters.

When the Romans brought the luxury of this Eastern bathing ritual to their own country, they gave these rooms names which are still used in steam baths today: tepidarium, caldarium, and laconicum; the cold room, or frigidarium, is sometimes just a basin of cold water or a plunge pool. A steam bath is ideal after a swim, beneficial to both mind and body, and incredibly luxurious if you give yourself the time to do it properly. Michelle, my beauty therapist, who is quite demanding and knowledgable describes an authentic steam bath that she experienced on a trip to Marmara in Turkey:

'I had the relaxing sensation of entering a series of immaculately clean, beautifully decorated marble and mosaic-tiled rooms, hearing the sound of trickling water from fountains, while men and women (in bathing suits) wandered from the tepid to the hot and then very hot steam rooms. After a time, having sweated a great deal, I was invited into another room and to lie on a marble slab where I was scrubbed down mercilessly, then sluiced off and wrapped in thirsty towels. I felt incredibly glowing and healthy. There was no rushing about. You could sit down afterwards and sip tea or a cool drink in another room until you felt like getting dressed and re-entering the world outside.'

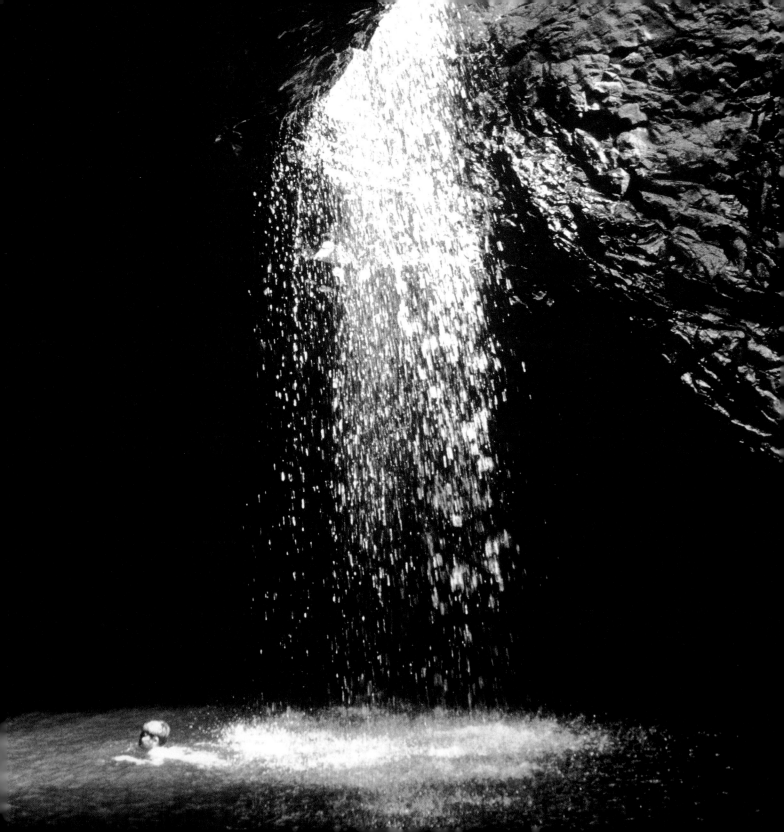

This sounds like an ideal way to initiate yourself to a steam bath, but if Turkey is too far to go for the day, see if your club or spa has a steam facility. A steam cabinet will not be as pleasurable as a steam room. Either way, however, you will gain the benefit of flushing the toxins from your skin and relaxing after your swim.

WILD SWIMMING

I grew up swimming in tame places, all of them civilised or supervised in some way. Even when I swam in the sea there was always a lifeguard present. I never had heard the wonderful expression 'wild swimming' before the publication of Roger Deakin's book *Waterlog*. Reading it reminded me of my most memorable swim – my wild swim.

It was on the spur of the moment in the clear, cold waters of a steep-walled, rocky gorge in central Australia on a hot, cloudless day. I had just landed that morning in Alice Springs and then driven for two and a half hours to this particular place which I had read about and was determined to see. The site was unspoiled, primeval. The trees, rocks and water were entrancing and before long I found myself longing to dive into the natural pool. There wasn't a soul around. You could hear the cry of a bird, nothing else, and as I entered the waters I felt that I had melted into the cool, limpid centre of the world.

The first pool was large, but I swam easily to its far side. This brought me to the gorge, ancient-looking, dark red rock, split to form a narrow, high-walled, secret-looking passage. I remember being able to touch both walls with my hands. High above me the sky was an intense blue.

I hesitated, then swam through it. The passage opened out into a magical series of pools, and then into another large, open lake. This was truly unknown country to me, and the swim was madness. I am not brave in that Raiders of the Lost Ark kind of way, but the magic of the setting, the clarity of the water, the sheer frisson of discovery led me on... And I was swimming so easily and well! Never had I felt so at one with nature, and, in fact, the universe.

Suddenly, three people seemed to appear from nowhere, from pools beyond mine, and as they came paddling towards me they were screaming, their high-pitched voices bouncing off the stony walls of the gorge. 'Swim back to shore!' they shouted, 'swim back to shore!' Did they own this magical, rock-bound gorge? 'Water snakes!' they hissed breathlessly, as they approached and then scooted past me on their sturdy airbeds. I had no airbed. In fact, since I had not planned on swimming at all, I was wearing nothing. 'They're poisonous! Swim back to shore – quick!' Suddenly I felt sick with a fear I had not known possible, my easy breathing started coming in short spurts and my arms and legs began churning up the calm, clear waters like a faulty outboard motor. In my mad frenzy to swim to shore, I was using every stroke I knew – all at the same time. Never had I swum so badly in my life! Yes, I made it back through the narrow gorge, (no, the people on the airbeds did not offer me transport). Finally I crawled out onto the shore and flopped down, safe, exhausted, my heart pounding. Call me a coward, but never again would I swim in unknown waters, certainly not in Australia.

Yet, that one swim was unforgettable. Roger Deakin sums up the sensation perfectly: 'When you swim, you feel your body for what it mostly is – water – and it begins to move with the water around it. To swim is to experience how it was before you were born.'

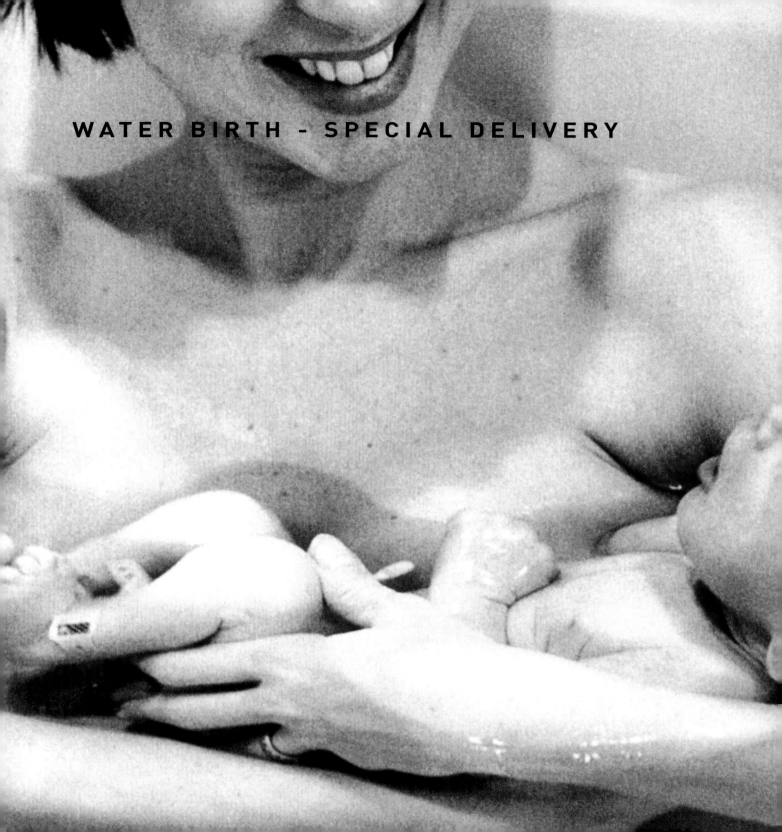

WATER BIRTH - SPECIAL DELIVERY

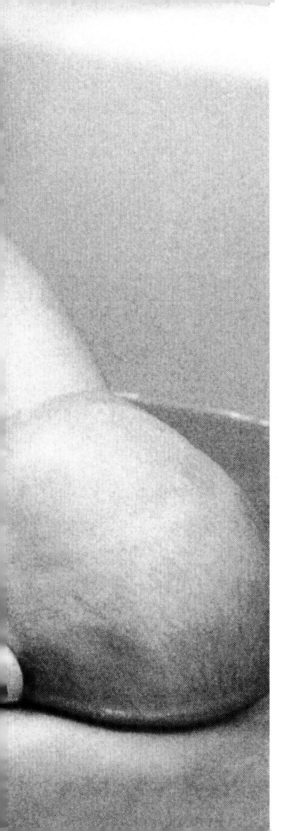

'Water, is taught by thirst.
Land – by the Oceans passed.
Transport – by throe –
Peace – by its battles told –
Love, by Memorial Mold –
Birds, by the snow.

EMILY DICKINSON

> The idea of giving birth in water is appealing because it sounds both logical and gentle. It is a form of hydrotherapy – there for you when you need it most. You lie back in a shallow pool of warm water, usually supported in some way. The warm water relaxes your muscles, easing back pain as well as the pain of the contractions. Mothers say that babies born this way seem calmer from the start.

'Giving birth' rather than 'being delivered' is the way most women would like to think of the experience of childbirth, whether you choose to have your baby at home or in hospital, in or out of water. The idea of giving birth in water is appealing because it sounds both logical and gentle. It is a form of hydrotherapy – there for you when you need it most. You lie back in a shallow pool of warm water, usually supported in some way. The warm water relaxes your muscles, easing back pain as well as the pain of the contractions. Mothers say that babies born this way seem calmer from the start.

Water birthing is probably as old as life itself, but as a technique it was pioneered in 1962 in the former Soviet Union by Igor Charkovsky, the male midwife and healer/shaman. He believed that conventional birthing methods disturbed the baby's delicate brain cells, whereas easing your baby into water keeps the brain cells in place and vibrant. Though there is no scientific evidence for Charkovsky's claims, he further suggested that water birthing heightens babies' abilities to access the world of psychic and paranormal experiences. The medical profession as a whole was not especially keen to pursue water birthing, but Charkovsky's methods were picked up enthusiastically by a few doctors, notably the French doctor Dr Michel Odent. He did a great deal to popularise and make possible water birthing from 1978 to 1985, and

gradually more and more women in Europe and America have been drawn to this method.

From the personal accounts I have heard and read, water birthing seems better for both mother and baby. Your baby exchanges its safe world of amniotic fluid for the warm and welcoming waters of the birthing tub. As your baby is born into the welcoming warm waters, the umbilical cord is cut and seconds later the baby 'swims' into your arms.

Water birthing is not as hard to arrange as it used to be, but not every hospital has the facilities. Whether you live in a major city or somewhere more rural, you have to pre-arrange a water birth to make it possible. In the UK, for example, you cannot just appear on the day with a 2m pool in tow and expect the hospital to welcome you! It is wise, wherever you live, to do some homework so you can organise a home or hospital water birth. Of course, if you go privately, it is easier to arrange.

If you are contemplating this way of giving birth, you probably have lots of questions. As well as asking your friends, doctor or local midwife for information, there are two organisations which offer help on a variety of levels, from simply answering your questions to arranging and facilitating the birth of your baby, from pre-natal to after-care help.

In the UK, the Birth Centre Ltd (tel: 020 7498 2322 or visit the website at www.birthcentre.com) offers a free, no-obligation consultation and can provide information on all aspects of birthing, not only water birthing, though the latter constitutes one third of the births the centre arranges. Whether or not you decide to use the services of the Birth Centre to have your baby, it can help you assess the choices available to you. It also offers an 'out of London' package, designed to link its care with that of your local midwife. You can have your baby at the Birth Centre, then return home where you can be looked after by your midwife, all of which the centre can help you arrange. This is only one of many packages offered by the centre, whose director, Professor Caroline Flint, RGN, RM, ADM, is past president of the Royal College of Midwives and author of five books for midwives and over 300 articles.

In the USA, the Global Maternal/Child Health Association (GMCHA) is focused wholly on water birthing (tel: 00 1 (503) 682 3600; website waterbirth@aol.com). It has been working for nearly ten years 'to preserve, protect, and enhance the well-being of women and children during pregnancy, birth, infancy and early childhood by educating practitioners, referring couples to practitioners, and helping couples take a portable tub into their local hospitals for labour or birth'. The association welcomes your questions.

Useful links from this website will help you with books to read and people to talk to who have given birth in water. *The Water Birth Handbook* by Dr Roger Lichy and Eileen Hertzberg is one to start with.

Another useful website is www.waterbirth.com which offers you background information and links you to sites for water birth classes and other resources.

Three of the questions most frequently asked about water birthing are considered below.

How does the baby breathe?

This is perhaps the most common question, stemming from the notion that the baby is under water for some time. The term 'under water birthing' as water birthing is also called, has probably given rise to this concern. In fact, as soon as your baby has fully emerged, someone – it could be you yourself, the baby's father, the midwife or the doctor – reaches down and gently hands your newborn to you. Until the moment when it is lifted out of the water, the baby is receiving its oxygen from you via the placenta and the umbilical cord. There is a complex physiological mechanism which keeps the baby from breathing when it is born in water, and it seems that the stimulus to breathe is from the baby's face coming into contact with air.

How hot should the water be?

The water should be at a comfortable temperature – between 32 and 38°C (90 and 101°F) because if it is too hot it could cause the baby's heart rate to rise. Keep handy some cold, wet face flannels or a spray bottle filled with cold water to refresh your baby – and yourself. (Charkovsky believed in dousing the heads of newborns with ice-cold water, so that the brain cells would first constrict, then expand. This rigorous custom was also practised by the Vikings!)

What is giving birth in water really like?

How does the experience of water birthing compare to 'ordinary' birthing? Is there really less pain? Is it just hype? Not everyone tells the truth about the pain of childbirth – or is it that they simply forget what it's like? This was the experience of my close friend Jane, who gave birth nine years ago to her son (and my godson) Joe, a confident, delightful, sensitive boy. It could be just a coincidence, but Joe is an excellent swimmer, loves to fish and, though he shows no signs as yet of being psychic, is brilliant with animals:

'I thought about the birth process and the alternatives available quite seriously with my second child. My first labour had been quick (four hours) and absolutely straightforward. I had a few gulps of gas and air but otherwise no intervention. I had the same marvellous midwife throughout the labour and birth. The only part of the experience that had been unpleasant was the fact that after each contraction, your limbs go shaky and weak as the contraction passes. Lying on a high bed, I had felt vulnerable and had worried about falling. It did not feel the right place to be.

My second child spent most of his time in utero in the breech position (feet, rather than head, down). As this can cause problems if the baby doesn't turn round before birth, I consulted a midwife from the Birth Centre to get all the information about breech births.

I also talked to them about water birth. I knew that the wonderful West London Hospital where I was going (now sadly closed) had a birthing pool and suddenly the image of lying supported in warm water seemed just right. I realised that the frightening trembling of limbs would be soothed away lying like that, so I put my name down for the pool when the time came.

Joe had done a timely somersault and had got himself into the right birth position and when we rang the hospital after my waters broke to say that we were coming in, the pool was free. I knew it was what I wanted and was really impatient to get in there in case someone else arrived and beat me to it!

It was just as delightful as I had imagined. The pool was about 2m long and 1m wide and was filled with warm water to a depth of about 60cm – enough to float comfortably. When my contractions started, I climbed in and lay back supported by a large rubber ring under my arms. It had a summery pattern of airborne seagulls on it. I was in a very comfortable position. The pain of the contractions came and then went at once, and I was able to relax deeply between them without the distressing shaking. The water buoyed me up.

I was naked, which felt right, and the body heat temperature seemed to dissolve my boundaries. I was in labour in the bath for about an hour and a half and then suddenly went into the second stage of labour and was overcome by the need to push. The midwife went to get a nurse as they seemed to require two for a water birth and after ten minutes Joe was born in two mighty heaves and was fished out and landed on the rubber ring round my chest. I looked at him and thought, 'He's just like a frog'. I am sure it must have been an easier journey for him to swim out of the womb into his mother's arms rather than have to be hauled into the air on the edge of a bed. My husband cut the cord, the midwife wrapped Joe in a blanket, I climbed out and lay on a bed. Joe and I had a cuddle and the nurse made some tea and toast. The entire experience was calm and natural and I don't think that this was at all to do with being more relaxed, as Joe is my second child.'

I am sure it must have been an
easier journey for him to swim out of
the womb into his mother's arms

WATERING YOUR SOUL

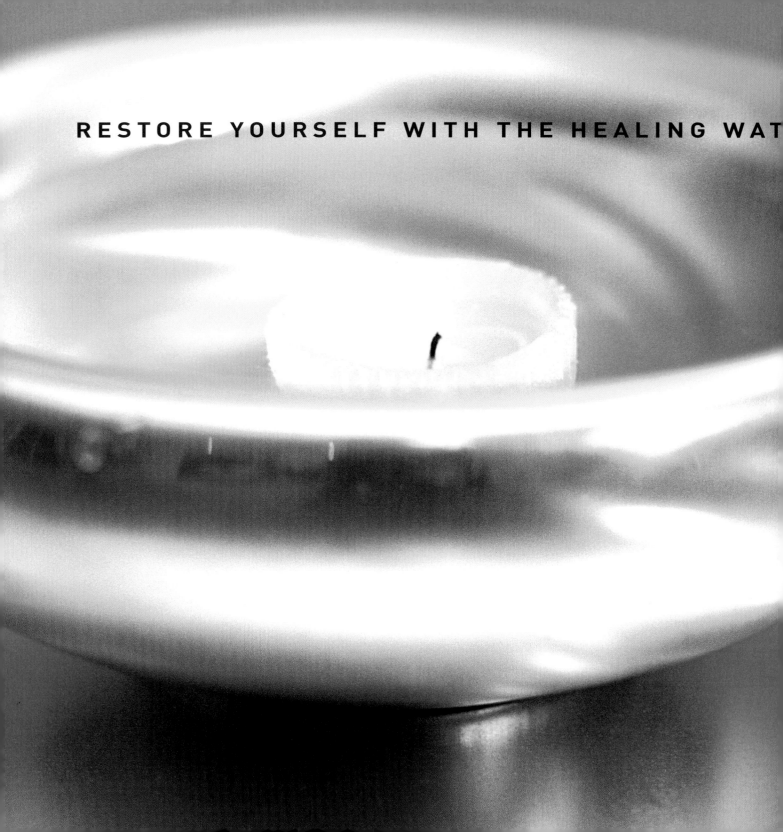

RESTORE YOURSELF WITH THE HEALING WAT

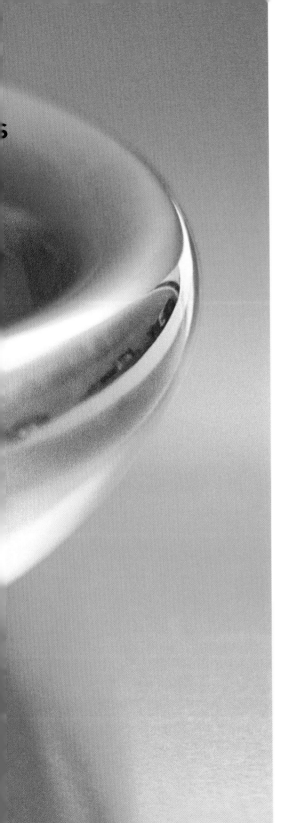

And the same night there fell a shower of rain,

For which their mouths gaped, like the cracks of earth

When dried to summer dust; till taught by pain,

Men really know not what good water's worth;

If you had been in Turkey or in Spain,

Or with a famish'd boat's-crew had your berth,

Or in the desert heard the camel's bell,

You'd wish yourself where truth is – in a well.

LORD BYRON
FROM DON JUAN, CANTO THE SECOND

We have always looked to natural water sources to heal not just our body but also our soul, from the purifying ritual baths of the ancient Greeks and Egyptians, to Lourdes' spring of miracles, to a reviving walk you or I might take today along the seashore. In ancient times, body and spirit were considered one. Heal one, heal the other. Cleansing your body with water was considered an integral part of the process of attaining purity of spirit – you were watering your soul as you watered your body.

Now this holistic approach is once more gaining acceptance, even by doctors and scientists who just a few years ago scoffed at the idea of any curative process that could not be measured and weighed, touched with the hand and seen by the eye.

We come from water. The creatures we're descended from began as infinitesimal, single-cell structures with a composition remarkably similar to that of our own cells. From creatures which crawled out of the sea hundreds of millions of years ago to our more recognisable earliest ancestors, *homo erectus*, the basic processes of the life function are inextricably dependent on water. It is no accident that on the shores of Lake Turkana, that huge expanse of water in the Great Rift Valley in Africa, the anthropologist Richard Leakey made his great discovery of the traces of early man.

'We are people of the lake,' he said. Our journey from that past is a long one, and each of us carries something from our collective past deep in our instinctive memory. Many believe that water itself has a 'memory'. Perhaps that is why sacred places and waterborne methods of spiritual renewal uniquely restore us. We live in a sceptical yet spiritually hungry age. More than ever we need to understand fresh and classic sources of renewal. From the magic of Delphi to the mass-immersions of the Ganges to the Feng-Shui simplicity of a garden fountain, water restores the human spirit every day.

Somewhere close by is a source that will restore yours.

RESTORE YOURSELF WITH THE HEALING WATERS SPRINGING UP THROUGHOUT THE WORLD

Why does water suddenly appear in one place, but not another? Why to this person and not to that? When will the rains come again – *if ever*? All these persistent and life-threatening questions meant that for centuries, water was both worshipped and feared. Precisely the unaccountability of water bestowed on it great mystery and magic. The sea, of course, was truly terrifying. Boats set out to sea and disappeared! Aristotle believed that creatures could die only at ebb tide. And this belief continued right up until the time of Shakespeare, who makes Falstaff die 'even just between twelve and one, even at the turning of the tide'. Springs, streams and the smaller rivers and lakes were not only life-giving, they were also contained within limits you could see, so fresh rather than saltwater sites became sacred. And however mysterious the sources, the meanings they were invested with were benign.

What if you could learn the secrets of water, make sense of its apparently capricious actions? Perhaps you could cure your illness, save your baby from original sin, even predict the future.

Journey with me to five sacred places, Delphi, Epidaurus,

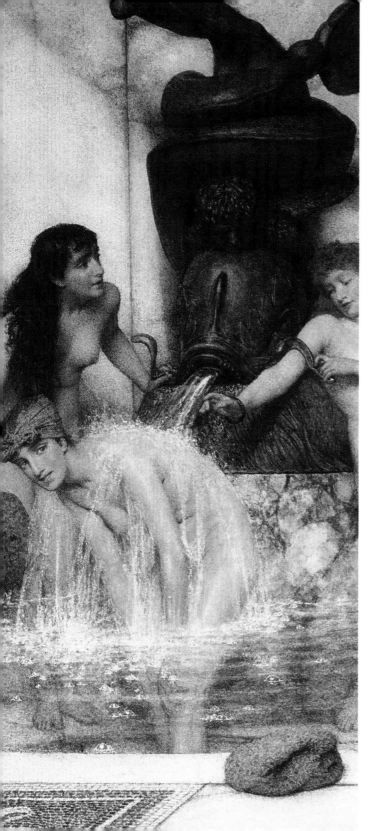

the Ganges, Lourdes and Glastonbury, and see how your spirit might be restored. Perhaps if you listen very carefully, you will hear your fate being whispered by water tumbling insistently, ceaselessly over rocks...

JOURNEY TO DELPHI: THE FOUNTAIN OF FATE

This most famous place of prophesy is one of the most extraordinary sacred sites of history. The ancient Greeks considered it the centre of the world and called it the 'omfalos gis', the navel of the earth. If you have never been, go there. Delphi rests amidst breathtaking mountain scenery near the Gulf of Corinth and owes its position, prominence and method of prophecy to the existence of fresh running water.

Between the cleft of two rocks which reflect the light, known as the Shining Rocks, is a precipice over 250 m (820 ft) high from which the locals used to hurl those found guilty of sacrilege. However, if you were wise enough to purify yourself in the Castalian Fountain which was fed from the mountain spring, presumably you were safe from any such accusations. In fact, anyone who came to Delphi for a religious purpose had first to purify himself – no women were permitted, except, of course for the Pythia, the priestess who delivered the oracle. This most important role was always reserved for a peasant woman over fifty years old. At the height of the oracle's fame there were three such priestesses.

Just like those who came to seek guidance, the priestesses also had to purify themselves in the Castalian Fountain, drink the water of the Kassotis and munch a laurel leaf from the bush by the fountain which Apollo had planted – myth and history being intertwined as ever. Only then could the priestesses take their seats on a kind of tripod, which was placed somewhat precipitously over a chasm, and from there

watering your soul   125

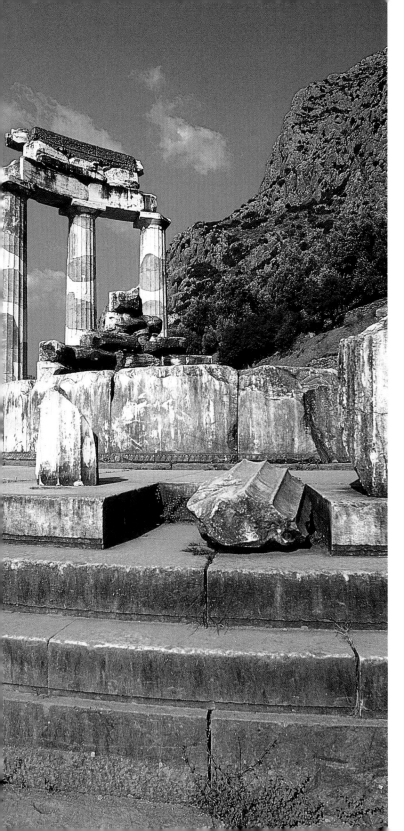

pronounce their often riddle-like predictions.

Perhaps the most famous, or notorious, of Delphic answers was made to King Croesus. He was a great benefactor of Delphi: perhaps he thought this would improve his fate? When he asked about the outcome of his planned war against Persia, the oracle said: 'If you attack Persia, a great empire will fall.' Delighted, Croesus led his army into battle, was defeated and lost his kingdom. What hadn't occurred to him was that the doomed 'great empire' could be his own.

For those who came to consult the oracle, the bathing of the hair in the Castalian Fountain was the principle part of the purification ceremony, prior to an audience with the priestess. Murderers, apparently, bathed the whole body.

At the base of the Castalian Fountain is a statue of Ge (or Gaia in Latin), the goddess of Earth, which indicates that the spring was an early place of cult worship. The spring itself was ornamented with a facade of seven marble pilasters, with niches for votive offerings. The water was collected in a long, narrow reservoir which fed seven jets. These jets fell into a rectangular court, reached by rock-hewn steps. The oracle drew streams of supplicants from all over the ancient world until it was finally abolished by the Christian Emperor Theodosius in about AD385. But people said that long before its extinction the oracle had become diminished, dealing in trivialities. Now the waters from the Castalian Fountain have been piped and you can drink them or take home a bottle: you can drink and cleanse yourself at the same water source used by people who journeyed there over two thousand years ago.

The overflow from the fountain eventually joins the waters of the spectacular gorge dividing the Phaedriades. This in turn plunges into a deep, rocky glen and merges with the

Pleistos river that flows in the Delphic valley far below. The oracles have ceased but the water's journey goes on and on. And whatever your opinions about soothsaying, ancient or modern, Delphi itself is unforgettable.

EPIDAURUS: THE ANCIENT GREEKS' HOLISTIC SPA

The Sanctuary of Asclepiades at Epidaurus was the most celebrated healing centre of the ancient world. Here, the healing waters were both spiritually and physically cleansing. Asclepiades was a physician so prominent he later was considered a god. Myth and history mingle, and he is on

courses of herbs to take for their lingering ills. There is no record of failures at the temple of Asclepiades but neither the chronically sick nor pregnant women were admitted which must have improved the statistics.

Epidaurus had a hospital, baths, the mineral spring, plus a sports area and a theatre which was renowned throughout the ancient world for its superb acoustics. Many of the famous Greek comedies were performed there. Laughter was, even then, the best medicine. Epidaurus was really an early spa: a combination of rest-cure, health resort and gym, with a bit of priestly psychotherapy thrown in. A 'miracle'

Epidaurus was really an early spa: a combination of rest-cure, health resort and gym, with a bit of priestly psychotherapy thrown in.

record as the father of two goddesses: Hygea, the goddess of health, from whose name comes the word 'hygiene', and Panacea, the goddess of remedies, whose name in turn is used to denote an all-healing or universal remedy.

Asclepiades' approach seems very modern today because it was holistic. At the heart of his system was the ritual of 'incubation' or temple sleep. Imagine yourself as a patient at Epidaurus, the largest of such centres. You would first bathe in the waters of the spring sacred to Asclepiades. The cleansing was intended to be both physical and spiritual. You would then lie down to sleep in one of the dormitories that adjoined the main part of the temple. As you slept, you would be visited in your dreams by Dr Asclepiades or by one of his priests who would advise you on what was wrong and what do about it. According to ancient records, many people would wake up cured. Others would be advised about diet or given

might well occur under these circumstances – perhaps with the aid of the kind of auto-suggestive techniques used in the incubation process. The priesthood was certainly skilled in its herbal and other ministrations. It is easy to see why the average stressed-out, over-taxed and over-indulgent ancient Greek would feel better after spending time here.

Epidaurus lies on an emerald-green, pine-fringed hill near the Gulf of Corinth. Like Delphi it is now a world heritage site, with a museum which includes many texts and artefacts relating to ancient Greek medicine. Many of the buildings have been restored. A trip to Epidaurus makes a wonderful day out from Athens, and a night at the open-air theatre is magic. But there is more to it than that. This is a place where you can close your eyes and imagine yourself bathing in clear waters, meditating and dreaming strange, healing dreams like those who travelled here so long ago.

BATHE IN THE GANGES: RIVER OF LIFE AND DEATH

The River Ganga in the north of India, known throughout most of the world by its anglicised name of Ganges, is perhaps the most sacred stretch of water on the face of the earth. And if you ever needed proof that the spiritually cleansing power of water is a phenomenon all of its own, go there. Because there you will see huge numbers of spiritually eager people bathing and praying and carrying out intimate and important rituals in what seems to a Westerner the most physically filthy environment imaginable.

The Ganges is one of seven sacred rivers in India. The others are the Yamuna, the Godavari, the Narmada, the Indus, the Cauvery, and the mythical Saraswati. There are many hundreds of places of pilgrimage in India, and many temples and pools where water plays a vital part in the process of spiritual purification. In fact, so key is the concept of water that the word tirtha – 'holy place', whether river or cave or mountain – means literally 'river ford'. All the same, the Ganges is considered especially holy. Its thousand-mile length, before it empties into the Bay of Bengal, is spotted with sacred sites said once to have witnessed crucial events in the incarnate lives of the great Hindu deities.

One of the most ancient and most-visited religious centres is the city of Varanasi (known to the British as Benares). At Varanasi the pilgrims come not only to gain spiritual refreshment and the strength to live life more fully, but also to die. Varanasi is sacred to the Hindu god Shiva (Sanskrit for 'Auspicious One'). It is perhaps typical of this fascinating, complex deity, for he combines the functions of restorer and destroyer, ascetic and sensualist, benevolent carer and wrathful avenger. In the last capacities, you might compare him to the Old Testament God, but the other qualities are uniquely Indian.

If you visit Varanasi, you will quickly find your way to the ghats, literally 'river steps', which lead down to the sacred Ganges itself. There are temples everywhere. All day the banks are full of sadhus ('holy men'), priests performing rituals, gurus teaching, pilgrims being blessed and praying and listening to wise words. People begin their ritual bathing at dawn, and the river grows more and more crowded as the day wears on.

Were you to enter the river, to wash yourself, to offer flowers or perhaps to light floating candles, you would emerge no cleaner than before, in fact possibly less so. The condition of your body would be no different, but you would be spiritually cleansed. The river water has no special mineral or physical properties. Nor, unlike at Epidaurus or the other great Graeco-Roman water sites, is the physical cleansing of the body relevant in any obvious sense.

At Varanasi sacredness of place is all.

Yet the fact that it's water in which the spiritual seekers choose to bathe is not meaningless. Flowing water is ever-changing and at the same time constant. It's vital for life, but can also kill. You cannot live in it, but you cannot live without it.

And at Varanasi, water's slow, shaping constancy meets its opposite element: fire. Fire's brief, destructive – or transforming – drama occurs here. Because of its sacredness to Shiva, many Hindus believe that to be cremated at Varanasi is to gain assurance of being reborn at a much higher level, or even of attaining the final emancipation which is the aim of the soul's religious journey. Both Mrs Indira Gandhi and her son Rajiv, recent prime ministers of India who fell victim to assassins, were cremated here, with fit ceremony. Other Hindus achieve this goal by dying here, or at least nearby, or perhaps in one of the many hospitals for incurable diseases in the city. Corpses are transported to the river by relatives, by truck, by taxi, even by rickshaw.

The 'burning ghat' is the special area where terraces of wood-fires burn the dead, who are dressed in sacred robes of bright yellow. The cremation rites are overseen by attendants who maintain the fires and, if necessary, ensure that the bodies are consumed by guiding the limbs to the fire with bamboo poles. Such a cremation is quite costly – about 5,000 rupees ($150 US, approx £70) – but the fires are kept busy twenty-four hours a day, every day of the year. Afterwards the ashes of the dead are scattered on the river. It all seems to many westerners astonishingly matter-of-fact, even callous. But meanwhile the pilgrims bathe and pray and rejoice.

While in the West we are rightly concerned to live well and fully, and to look after our health and our appearance, we tend to confine ourselves to a disinfected, cosseted world where the big issues are rarely confronted and the dead hardly ever seen. The Hindu pilgrim bathing in the Ganges has more important things to think about than hygiene – such as the purification of the soul. And within his or her sight, the dead undergo their final, drastic transformation by fire. Then they are consigned not just literally to the waters of the Ganges but also metaphorically to the eternal, ever-flowing river that is synonymous with life and time.

WITNESS LOURDES, THE SPRING OF MIRACLES

Lourdes is a place about which it is easy to be sceptical, even cynical. This Catholic religious site welcomes five million visitors a year and rivals Mecca as a place of pilgrimage. If you go, you fly into its own airport and stay nearby in one of 350 hotels. Lourdes is so famous it even has the privilege of a

pop icon, Madonna, giving her daughter its name. Perhaps Madonna (herself named after the Virgin Mary) is sincere in her rediscovered faith, and perhaps there is good reason why this picturesque but relatively undistinguished town at the foot of the Pyrenees has attracted tens of millions of pilgrims during the past 140 years.

The story of how this came about is an extraordinary one. Bernadette Soubirous, a fourteen-year-old miller's daughter, was collecting firewood one February day in 1858, when she claimed to have met the Virgin Mary who revealed to her the source of a curative spring. There began its reputation as the healing place of the Western world, a byword for desperate, last-chance treatment and miraculous recovery.

Most people know the story from the Hollywood film The Song of Bernadette. This is based on a novel by the German-Jewish writer Franz Werfel, a fervent anti-Nazi and humanitarian. Werfel had been forced to flee first to France and then, when Hitler's armies moved in, to the South of France. There, though still in danger from the collaborationist authorities, he could plan his escape from Europe. For some time he stayed at Lourdes, already an internationally known religious site. A sophisticated man inclined to scepticism, he nonetheless found himself surrounded by such an atmosphere of kindness and goodness that he became persuaded that the town really must be a special place. When he finally reached safety in America, he wrote the novel on which the Hollywood film was based.

It seems impossible to deny that between February and July 1858, Bernadette experienced a series of visions of the Virgin Mary. Bernadette's family had fallen on hard times and they lived in miserable conditions. Her health had been damaged by a childhood bout of cholera and she suffered from continuing health problems which were to carry her off at the age of thirty-five. Many believe that her 'encounter' was the product of a fevered hallucination.

Yet the persistence of this shy, sickly child was extraordinary. She stuck to her account of her meeting with the Virgin in the face of aggressive scepticism from the law, the state and most of the church authorities. And over the years that followed, the spring which Bernadette said she had discovered, by scratching in the ground at the behest of the Blessed Virgin, became a place of pilgrimage, first for a few, and then – when miracles started happening – for increasing numbers of sick and despairing people. This is the spring which is at the heart of the by now huge Lourdes complex, and it is here that 400,000 people – including 70,000 seriously ill or disabled visitors bathe every year.

Since 1858 thousands of cures have been claimed. Yet a total of only sixty-five (sixteen since the end of the Second World War) have been certified as miracles by the Catholic Church-appointed committee of specialists. These specialists have in the past included Nobel laureates. How is 'miracle' defined in this case? As a long-term recovery from an identifiably incurable disease, such as cancer, multiple sclerosis, tuberculosis, blindness and paralysis. In other words, the cures cannot, so far as the committee could ascertain, have occurred other than through divine intervention. When you think about it, even one miracle is impressive; a real miracle every couple of years is truly astonishing.

The waters of Lourdes are found in the grotto near the River Pau, a lonely, inaccessible spot until Bernadette brought the Virgin's spring to life there. Now, of course, pilgrims crowd the paved boulevard, invalids throng the chilly blue marble baths, and at busy times visitors queue to fill bottles with water piped from the spring. For all this, there is one interesting fact that everyone involved admits: the waters of the Lourdes spring contain no discernible medicinal properties, not even mineral elements, that might possibly contribute to the 'cures' or the miracles. Faith and prayer are the ingredients. Lourdes' basilica holds seven thousand worshippers.

Faith and the prayer do not come cheap. You have to travel there and find somewhere to stay. Signs in the holy site explain why, when you buy a large candle, your prayers will 'last longer'. At night the neon signs of the hotels waiting to house the faithful can make the town feel more like Las Vegas than a holy shrine. You can even buy bottles of Lourdes Water on the internet ($45 for three including shipping), each incorporating a tasteful plastic statue of the Blessed Virgin. And yet...

A London doctor I know, sensible, sophisticated and undramatic, went years ago as a young intern to Lourdes with a group of fellow doctors to help the sick and the disabled. He went, like Werfel, as a sceptic. He took in all the tacky atmosphere as well as the obvious piety and the simple faith. He witnessed no dramatic cures and the experience did not return him to Catholicism. But what he saw and felt there was unforgettable. He came away with an understanding of how faith inspires people who ordinarily have no reason to hope. It was, he said, something larger than himself, than any one of us. When he talks about it now, thirty years later, you can see that it is as fresh and mysterious an experience as the spring water itself.

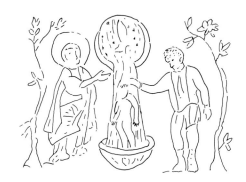

DIP YOUR BABY IN SACRED WATERS

The word 'baptism' comes from the Greek meaning 'to dip', and the idea of symbolising spiritual change by an act of immersion in water is extremely ancient, found almost everywhere in the world. As an eighteenth-century account states:

'Purification by washing was used in all the mysteries thousands of years before our era. In India, Persia, Egypt, and at Eleusis, initiates were always so purified... In every cavern of Salsette, in India, was a carved basin, to contain the consecrated water of ablution, used in initiation. In the mysteries of Mithras, in Persia, there were lavers (as it were of regeneration) in which the priest washed the neophytes, purifying them and symbolically expiating their sins. The followers of Zoroaster baptised children, as a token of purification of the soul...the Etruscans baptised with air, fire and water.'

The ancient Druids also carried out a rite of initiation involving the sprinkling of water on the heads of devotees. But the custom of baptising, and the pivotal significance attached to it as a life-changing experience, is particularly strong in the Christian tradition. And now the ceremony is associated almost wholly with the reception of infants (and sometimes adults) into the Christian church. Is there, then, any difference between the Christian ceremony and these even more ancient practices? Christians think so, of course. St John Chrysostom, fourth-century Greek patriarch and archbishop of Constantinople, wrote of baptism: 'It represents death and burial, life and resurrection... When we plunge our head into water as into a tomb, the old man is immersed, wholly buried; when we come out of the water, the new man appears at that moment.'

So baptism is not just a metaphorical purification but a rebirth. Its presence in Christian ritual, right from the start, is accounted for by most authorities as coming more or less directly from Jewish rituals. Most obvious of these is the *mikvah*, the cleansing ritual bath used by women, especially post-menstrually, but there were also ritual baths involved in ceremonies of conversion, accompanied by certain prayers. John the Baptist's use of immersion ceremonies in the River Jordan as part of his ritual of discipleship – this was where he baptised Jesus – may or may not have come from mainstream Jewish ritual. There is evidence that John was a member of the Essenes, a Jewish monastic sect whose initiation rituals included a form of baptism (as we know from the Dead Sea scrolls, which were Essene documents).

There is nevertheless disagreement about whether Jesus himself ordained baptism, full immersion in water, during his lifetime as a rite of acceptance into his spiritual circle. The solitary explicit mention comes in Matthew's gospel, where the Risen Christ exhorts his disciples to 'go therefore and make disciples of all nations, baptising them in the name of the father and of the son and of the holy spirit, teaching them to observe all that I have commanded you'.

Certainly baptism became widespread very early in the

history of Christianity. It is described in the Acts of the Apostles, and just a few decades after Jesus's crucifixion St Paul compared baptismal immersion to sharing in the death, burial, and resurrection of Christ. This is the key element that distinguishes Christian baptism from other purification or lustration rituals: it does not merely cleanse but also commits the person who undergoes it to a very specific and possibly arduous spiritual journey. Hence the arguments over the centuries among theologians about whether a baby, a creature incapable of rational choice, can actually be baptised.

Radical groups such as the sixteenth-century Anabaptists practised only adult baptism, as do many other Protestant sects of today. Meanwhile, mainstream Christianity came up with the idea of Confirmation, where, having been provisionally received into the church at birth, the individual on the threshold of adult life 'tops up' the baptismal commitment with a conscious reaffirmation. (Oddly, the Greek Orthodox Church, into which I was born, combines baptism and confirmation in one ceremony when you are an infant and far too young to 'confirm' anything.)

Many critics, including feminists, have claimed that Christian baptism, far from being a spiritually uplifting process, was rapidly turned by its patriarchal creators into a dark denial of life. In *The Woman's Encyclopaedia of Myths and Secrets*, Barbara G. Walker points to the decision by the church in AD 418 to treat the unbaptised child as inherently evil:

'The church's teaching was that every new-born infant before baptism belonged to the Devil. St Augustine's doctrine of original sin laid the foundation for this idea, and Tertullian said that every baby was born evil; its soul is 'unclean' and 'actively sinful' before baptism. Medieval theologians held that any infant still in the womb is doomed to damnation.'

Of course, few modern theologians outside the fundamentalist fringe would claim any such thing these days, as Walker admits.

Why would anyone baptise their baby today? I doubt whether any parents believe that their baby is heading for damnation unless it is sprinkled with water. But that does not completely destroy the point of baptism. You might want to provide your new-born child with a ceremony that welcomes him or her into the life of your family and the community. Your friends and relatives will be there to support your child as he or she progresses along the possibly rocky road to adulthood. And if you are a Christian, or believe in Christian precepts as a guide to living, why not hold that ceremony in a church?

Many folk-myths detail ways of safeguarding a child in its new-born, unformed state – in other words, until that family and community support system groups around it. In the Scottish Hebrides, it's said there are still clear remnants of pre-Christian ritual in the habit of carrying a torch around the baby's cradle each day, to keep it safe until baptism. In the Baltic state of Estonia, country people will not say the baby's name out loud before it is pronounced at the baptismal ceremony – for fear that until then the Devil, if he knows it, will seize the child's unprotected soul.

Water, whether in a river, pool or font, or symbolically sprinkled over the child, cleanses and protects, as it has for thousands of years. Immersion as a metaphor for renewal is as old as humankind.

DISCOVER THE HOLY WELL OF HEALTH

Christianity has taken the place of many established and ancient religious systems. When it could not suppress them, it tried to absorb aspects of these 'pagan' beliefs into its own body of ritual. So, for example, in Africa, as well as in the African-influenced Caribbean and in Brazil, we find elements of voodoo and animist traditions in the church's worship. In Mexico, ceremonies such as the Day of the Dead clearly reflect the ancestor- and death-worship that was a strong part of Mayan and Aztec religion. Throughout Western Europe, especially where Celtic people lived, the most stubborn remnants of the 'old religion' survive in water-worship, including the veneration of wells and pools as sources of fertility and healing.

It was this area of religious practice that the church decided to tolerate, and even to celebrate. Around AD 600 it became policy to rename pagan wells after Christian saints, so that any powers they might be invested with would thereby become respectable. Christian saints were given credit for any beneficial effects.

A hundred years ago a traveller in the British Isles wrote:

'The stranger in Ireland, or the Highlands of Scotland, hears rumours of a distinguished well, mile on miles off. He thinks he will find an ancient edifice over it, or some other conspicuous adjunct. Nothing of the kind. He has been lured all that distance, over rock and bog, to see tiny spring bubbling out of the rock, such as he may see hundreds of in a tolerable walk any day. Yet, if he search in old topographical authorities, he will find that the little well has ever been an important feature of the district; that century after century it has been unforgotten...'

Of course, the veneration of water was and is not unique to the British Isles or even Western Europe. At Mecca, holiest of Islam's holy places, there is a sacred spring at which pilgrims ritually wash themselves. Throughout North America, the predominantly animist native population revered all sources of water, however apparently minor. But Christianity presents a spectacular example of positive and ultimately rewarding adaptation. A surprising number of major religious sites in Western Europe are centred around sources of water which may have pre-Christian significance.

There are countless examples. The famous cathedral of St James at Santiago do Campostela in north-western Spain is, after Rome and Lourdes, the third most revered destination for Christian pilgrims. No mention of the fact is made in modern guidebooks, but medieval accounts assert that the cathedral altar was built directly over an ancient spring. The cathedrals of Chartres and Notre Dame are also placed over even older religious sites – Notre Dame de Paris on an island in the Seine used first for Druidic water rituals and then by the Romans as a temple of Jupiter.

In Britain and Ireland the coincidence is near-universal, as the church deliberately positioned its houses of worship over pre-Christian sites. So many English churches have holy wells, often suspected to be of pagan provenance, 'in their basements'. These include grand foundations such as York Minster, Carlisle Cathedral, Winchester Cathedral, Walsingham Abbey, and the famous London churches of St Bride's and St Olav's, as well as hundreds of ordinary parish churches.

The water from these wells was often used in baptisms. And all these places were visited during the so-called Dark Ages and in medieval times by people seeking divine intervention to cure disease or infertility. After all, where was the conventional medicine that might help them, especially the masses of peasants and labourers and their families?

But pilgrimage to such sights was not confined to the poor and lowly. The English King Henry VIII, desperate for his first wife, Catherine of Aragon, to bear him a son, walked barefoot from London to the monastery church at Walsingham to pray at its holy well. It is said that his bitterness at the failure of his plea led to the English Reformation. It certainly seems true that the monks of Walsingham were especially harshly treated when the monasteries were dissolved.

Throughout northern Europe, the Reformation brought Protestant rigour and official discouragement of the kind of semi-heathen practices which the Catholic Church had tolerated out of respect for the common people's practical spiritual needs. In England this rarely translated into punitive action. In Scotland, though, the Kirk fined those who committed the 'crime' of visiting a holy well and in some places even physically destroyed the sites.

All the same, the custom continued in a sometimes covert fashion. In fact, even in Victorian times, wells were being used in a way that bore a startling resemblance to early Christian baptism. Janet and Colin Board's fascinating book *Sacred Waters* quotes an eyewitness from Wigtown, in the Scottish borders, describing a sick baby being 'treated' at a well:

'The child was stripped naked, and taken by the spaul – that is, by one of the legs – and plunged headforemost into the big well until completely submerged; it was then pulled out, and the part held on by was dipped in the middle well, and then the whole body was finished by washing the eyes in the smallest one… An offering was

then left in the old chapel, on a projecting stone inside the cave behind the west door, and the cure was complete.'

Since the 1960s the rise of the 'New Age' movement has led to increased interest in old holy wells, especially ones with pre-Christian or Druidic connections. Most fairly well-known wells are regularly visited. In some cases, people will collect water to use for baptisms and other rituals. In others, they will tie rags around branches and bushes at the site. This is a revival of the old ritual whereby supplicants at the well would 'transfer' their sickness to the cloth, which would then wither, taking the illness with it. (The word 'tawdry' arises from this practice because of an association with St Audrey and her torn garments.)

As the phenomenon that is Lourdes proves, faith is a powerful force and there is no explaining it. While we might accept that some wells could contain beneficial minerals, it seems unlikely that most have more than an ancient tradition, a beautiful site and a holy name to offer. Call it faith, the placebo effect, or just plain chance, but these places had and often continue to have a reputation for helping people from all walks of life recover from illness or unhappiness.

DRINK IN THE TRANQUILLITY OF THE CHALICE WELL

The spring that feeds the Chalice Well at Glastonbury has never failed and its waters are still used for baptism and healing. To enter this oasis of calm and drink the waters is to participate in a ritual going back at least two thousand years, though records only exist from AD 1200. Here, as in many sacred sites, history meets religion and myth.

The legend goes that after Christ's crucifixion, St Joseph

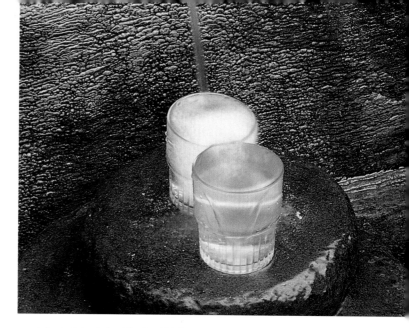

of Arimathea, the merchant disciple who took Jesus from the cross, travelled to Glastonbury, then an island settlement among treacherous coastal marshes (the 'Isle of Avalon'). It was there he chose to deposit the cup, or chalice, of the Last Supper. The well is said to have sprung into being when Joseph struck the ground with his staff (a common mythic explanation in all cultures for the origin of sacred springs is that a holy man brought it into being in this or a similar dramatic way). Some even suppose that the Druids, to whom the place was also sacred, welcomed the saint.

There is no hard evidence for any part of this story, but also no question that Glastonbury has been regarded as a sacred site since time immemorial. A Christian church has existed there since at least the second century AD, and the monastery that sprang from these beginnings had grown rich and powerful long before the end of the first millennium. Some accounts claim that Ireland's St Patrick ended his days here as abbot. Lack of historical records has not deterred countless pilgrims – from St Bridget in the fifth century to modern-day visitors – from flocking to Glastonbury.

Iron-rich water from the Mendip Hills colours the spring and the surrounding stones rusty red, which has led to an association with the blood of Christ, supposedly contained in the chalice. It is certainly true that the mineral content alone cannot explain the specific curative powers documented. That did not stop Dr John Dee, the illustrious Elizabethan mathematician and astrologer, from declaring in 1582 that he had found the 'Elixir Vitae' here. An eighteenth-century account relates how the waters cured a young gentleman of asthma, news which brought ten thousand people rushing to Glastonbury. Claimed cures of various ills included king's evil (tuberculosis of the lymph glands), blindness, ulcers and deafness.

I first visited the Chalice Well one hot and humid day in June. My head was jangling with schedules and deadlines. I was exhausted and – having read all the historical background – feeling more than a little sceptical. The well and its grounds nestle at the foot of Glastonbury Tor, which rises 100 m (330 ft) above the Somerset flatlands. There is a modest entrance fee, and visitors are encouraged not just to sample the waters but also to take some home. I walked among the beautifully terraced gardens, then sat on the lush green grass listening to the never-failing spring as people came and cupped their hands to drink from the lion's head fountain. Gradually, a tangible sense of calm began to quell my anxieties – and my sceptical, stress-fuelled thoughts. The healing power for me comes from the elemental combination of wood, water and stone found at so many sacred sites, from Delphi to Lourdes. The healthful presence of negative ions is a scientific explanation. Could it also be the result of some mysterious ingredient in the water itself? I know I felt profoundly restored and the way ahead seemed to untangle and become clear. My memory of that afternoon continues to refresh me.

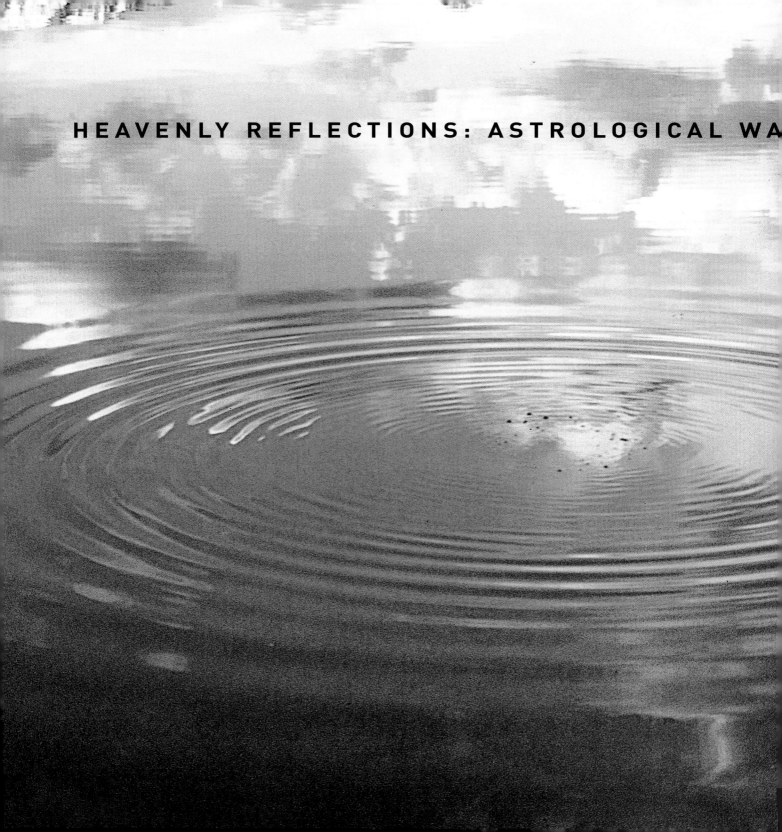

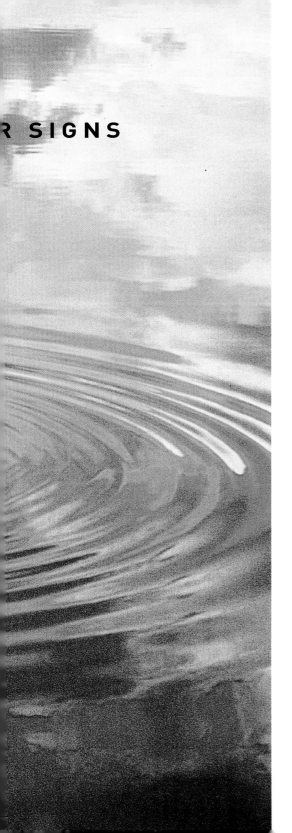

R SIGNS

'A lake is the landscape's most beautiful and expressive feature. It is earth's eye, looking into which the beholder measures the depth of his own nature.'

HENRY DAVID THOREAU

'Whatever is born or done at this moment of time has the qualities of this moment of time.' Professor Jung was a great psychologist with an intense interest in supposedly 'unscientific' ways of interpreting the world – including astrology. Perhaps a more familiar way of expressing what he means in this opening quotation is the much older adage 'As above, so below' – heavenly reality (or call it the abstract ideal) as reflected on earth. The Chinese philosophy of feng shui incorporates this principle when it codifies the balancing forces of the elements.

What astrology claims to do is to take a snapshot of the exact position of the universe at the time of your birth – no two individuals will have the same snapshot – and then project forward the movements, elements and constellations that will condition (not necessarily predict) the events of your life.

I am an intrigued sceptic when it comes to astrology. I always feel better if someone reads my fortune and predicts an excellent month ahead. But I don't believe it. On the other hand, I have been dazzled on two occasions by skilled practitioners who seemed to 'know me' and to understand my life. So there are really two worlds of astrologers – can anyone believe the hit-and-miss predictions of the tabloid entertainers who claim to be able to divide the world's population into twelve and forecast exactly what is going to happen to them over a given period in their future according to their sun-sign?

Of course, respectable astrologers such as Liz Greene (who also happens to be a qualified Jungian psychologist, and one of the people who dazzled me) never work with sun-signs alone. Nor is 'prediction' what she does. There are rising signs, moon-signs, aspects, conjunctions, a whole host of other factors which can be just as important in an individual's life and which are constantly changing. And there are the four elements, fire, earth, air and water.

According to classic astrology, the cycle of the zodiac begins with fire, which governs the signs of Aries, Leo and Sagittarius. All of these are dramatic, volatile, bright-burning. It continues with earth: the solid, real, orderly qualities of Capricorn, Taurus and Virgo. Then there is air; Aquarius, Gemini and Libra – intellectual, intangible, constantly striving to make sense of the world through the mind.

And finally water: Pisces, Cancer, and Scorpio. The element of fluidity and emotion which embraces the qualities of imagination, empathy and sensitivity. Think of the ocean, how it ebbs and flows, how its mood constantly changes, stormy then calm. A person born under the sign of water is able to adapt to and understand almost any situation and yet remain uncompromised and true to oneself. But, of course, the sun is not the only influence taken into account by serious astrologers. The quality of water is present in some aspect of you, even if your sun-sign makes you think of yourself as earthy, airy or fiery.

WATER SIGNIFIES THE FLOW OF FEELING

All astrologers seem to agree that the essence of the element of water is feeling, emotion and because of that, constant change. And yet, although always moving and changing shape, ebbing and flowing, as in the physical reality of water, it is always there. Although you might frequently be switching your mood, if water is strong in your sign, you tend

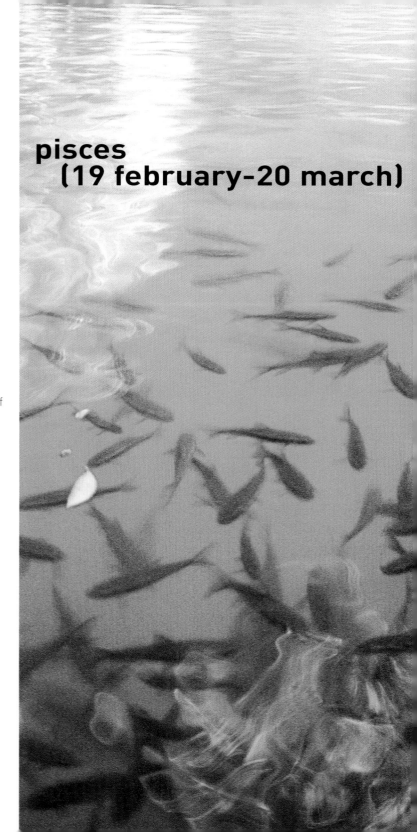

to be a person who is 'contained' in relationships, as Jung described it. You are the one who wants to be needed, so you therefore often provide the emotional underpinning to partners who are more inflexible, less sensitive and caring. Imagination, empathy and sensitivity define you.

If these sound like wonderful characteristics, they are – even if they don't always feel like it. People strongly influenced by this element overcome difficulties and dangers by flowing around and over them rather than facing them head-on. They make human relations easier, and water people in general are excellent in all people-orientated situations and professions.

FISHES, CRABS AND SCORPIONS IN THE SKY

The sun-signs in Western astrology traditionally represent where the sun is crossing the heavens during certain times of the astrological year. For the water signs this happens at the these three time of the year: at the end of winter (Pisces the Fish), in high summer (Cancer the Crab) and at the end of autumn (Scorpio the Scorpion). Any one or none of these signs may also have been ascendant or in some other position at that same time, affecting aspects of your personality or the complex set of circumstances to which we give the rather daunting name of 'fate'. So pay attention to all the characteristics of each sign, because no matter what your 'sun-sign' might be, they may well play a role in your life:

Pisces (19 February–20 March)

The symbol for Pisces is two fishes swimming in opposite directions – in the depths of the sea, where all is unpredictable and seemingly limitless. The sign was

pisces (19 february-20 march)

associated by the ancients with the god of the sea, Neptune – and by later seers with Christ, the fisher of men. Pisceans are endlessly curious, mystical, romantic. You swim and swim, scooping up everything in your way as if it were so much plankton, and (like real fish) you can be slippery,

master all of life, including the dark side. This may lead you into areas of passion and peril where others would fear to tread. Your emotional intensity can frighten others, though you are also capable of powerful love and great loyalty.

According to the flying stars system, the following are the water years of the twentieth century: 1909, 1918, 1927, 1936, 1945, 1954, 1963, 1972, 1981, 1990.

unreliable. Everything is important to you – and nothing. Einstein had Pisces as his sun-sign.

Cancer (21 June– 22 July)

This sign is symbolised by the crab, a creature at home both on the land and in water, the spheres of practical life and of the emotions. Unlike the Fish, you experience boundaries, represented by the secure shell into which you can withdraw when circumstances warrant. Also unlike the Fish, the Crab cares deeply about security. Therefore you are conservative and can appear secretive. But once sure of yourself, you are intuitive, affectionate, compassionate and public-spirited. Unlike the other water signs you also have an instinctive grasp of what is possible in business.

Scorpio (23 October–21 November)

As its name implies, this is the sign of the Scorpion, a desert animal that thrives at night and can retaliate in an extremely painful way if threatened. The Scorpion is also, however, a determined and resourceful creature which is supremely able to triumph over its dangerous environment. The feeling here is one of a fierce, almost savage will to

FLYING STARS

The Chinese organise their astrological calculations differently. Their flying stars – or 'nine-star ki' – is based on the I Ching, a three-thousand-year-old philosophy. To simplify the complex system of time-cycles within time-cycles ranging from 13,500 years to nine days, they associate an element with the year of birth of a person (or of a state, a relationship or a business). This explains the fortunes of these subjects and suggests what cures might be suitable when things go awry. The Chinese have five elements: earth, fire, wood, metal and water.

According to the flying stars system, the following are the water years of the twentieth century: 1909, 1918, 1927, 1936, 1945, 1954, 1963, 1972, 1981, 1990. Remember that the Chinese New Year starts later than the Western one: on the 4/5 February. So if you were born in January 1954, for example, you could not claim to have been born in a Water year, but if you were born at the same time in 1955, you could. Curiously a Water year did not occur in 1999 as you would expect from the previous sequence, or in 2000. In fact, water will not re-surface until after 2005. The unpredictability of water is the only explanation I can offer. Perhaps the first few years of the millennium won't be so emotional after all.

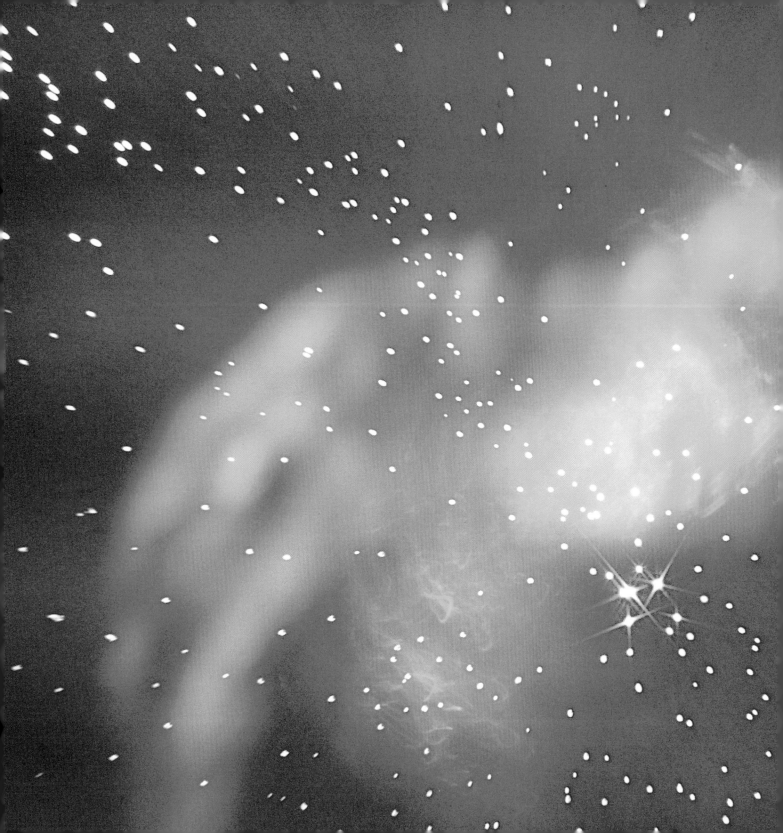

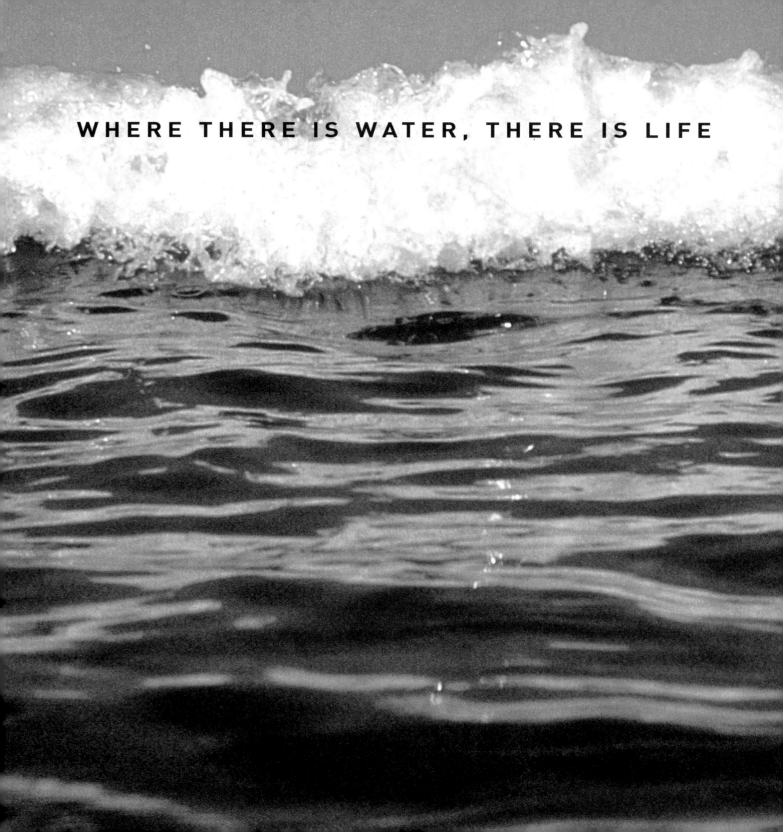

WHERE THERE IS WATER, THERE IS LIFE

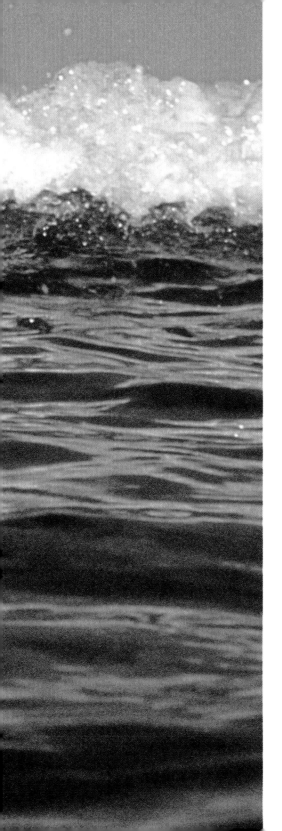

This celestial seascape with white herons got up as angels,
flying as high as they want and as far as they want sidewise
in tiers and tiers of immaculate reflections;
the whole region, from the highest heron
down to the weightless mangrove island
with bright green leaves edged neatly with bird droppings
like illumination in silver,
and down to the suggestively Gothic arches of the mangrove
roots

and the beautiful pea-green back-pasture
where occasionally a fish jumps, like a wild flower
in an ornamental spray of spray;
this cartoon by Raphael for a tapestry for a Pope:
it does look like heaven.
But a skeletal lighthouse standing there
in black and white clerical dress,
who lives on his nerves, thinks he knows better.
He thinks that hell rages below his iron feet,
that that is why the shallow water is so warm,
and he knows that heaven is not like this.
Heaven is not like flying or swimming,
but has something to do with blackness and a strong glare
and when it gets dark he will remember something
strongly worded to say on the subject.

ELIZABETH BISHOP
SEASCAPE

After a downpour the other day I ventured out into the dripping garden with my dog Calypso. The air and sky were rinsed clean. In the unexpected blaze of sunlight, every leaf, each blade of grass shone a bright, luminous green. The earthenware pot that sits by the door for Calypso to drink from was brimful with rainwater and she dipped her head eagerly towards it.

But instead of drinking she hesitated, sat down and simply stared, whimpering, into its depths. I knelt down to see what was stopping her. I could hear a swishing sound. Something was moving beneath the surface. As I looked closer, a pointy head with bulbous, half-lidded eyes suddenly came peering out at me over the rim and I could see the creature's lean little leathery arms and legs keeping up a frantic breast-stroke, fruitless against the large, slippery-sided pot.

As I cupped the struggling frog and carried it to our pond, its familiar habitat, I was reminded of the following haiku by the famous Japanese poet Bashō who wrote these timeless lines some five hundred years ago:

The old pond –
A diving frog.
The sound of water

Even a pot of water, I thought to myself, attracts life... Where there's water there is life. Its presence not only ensures life, it revives your spirit and refreshes your soul. In the following pages I suggest ways to help you recognise, create and keep a water source ever-present in your life so you can draw on it every day.

TAKE A WALK BY MOVING WATER

When you feel over-tired and stressed, you often cannot summon up the energy you need to regain your balance, your sense of well-being, even your sense of humour. Although you know there are simple, everyday things which would make you feel better, your creative spirit lies stagnant. If you resist overcoming that stagnation, you can find yourself spiralling into depression.

Whenever I feel low, I know that I feel cut off from my senses. My conscious feeling is that nothing much matters. To reconnect to something deep in myself I depend on nature. I walk along the beach. Every wave that breaks reminds me how good it is just to be alive. There's a scientific explanation for the heightened sense of well-being which moving water engenders. You might think it unromantic – after all, the beauty and power of the sea, a waterfall or a fast-flowing river should be reason enough to make you feel better. True, but knowing there is a scientific basis adds to rather than detracts from the pleasure and sense of connection which the sea inspires.

Polluted air or a stormy atmosphere contains positive ions which scientists believe depresses the brain's ability to release serotonin, the mood controller that makes you feel happy and energetic. (You might find that you get a headache when the barometer is dropping, which indicates that a storm

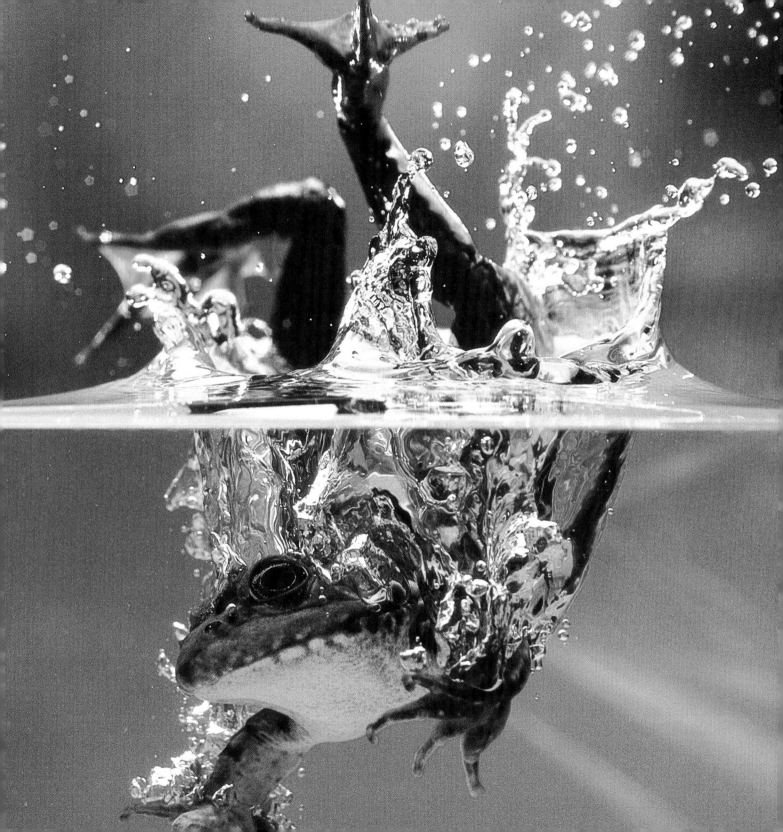

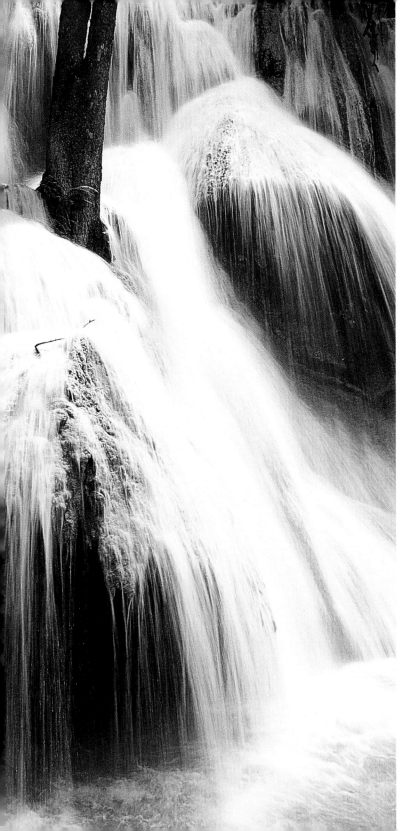

is imminent.) In contrast, water that is in motion releases a mass of negative ions. These negative ions fly free when, for example, the storm breaks and the rains finally come. Similarly, by the sea, when the waves are crashing and you feel the fine spray on your face, you are inhaling negatively charged air. So following a storm, at a waterfall or on the seashore, the air is always negatively charged and you feel terrific, or at least a whole lot better.

The feel-good factor is especially strong at Niagara Falls, the destination of countless honeymooners. Niagara, which lies on the border between the USA and Canada border, is a monumental concentration of negative ions – and not a bit overrated. Like Venice, though in a completely different way of course, its power and magnificence entirely live up to your expectations.

To the Iroquoian people of the north-east, the falls symbolised the victory of good over evil. The native American mythology relates how thunder hurled its lightning bolts at a monster water snake which had caused sickness and misery to a local Seneca village. The snake's dead body became lodged in the bedrock of the Niagara river, and so the waters pour over the spent evil force in the tumultuous, ceaseless cascade of this incredible waterfall. Go there and breathe in pure energy.

LEARN A LITTLE FENG SHUI: THE WAY OF WIND AND WATER

Feng shui (pronounced foong shway) translated means the way of wind and water. It is fundamentally based on the I Ching, a Chinese philosophy written some three thousand years ago by a sage called Fu Hsi. According to the Chinese legend, Fu Hsi was sitting beside the Lo river in northern

China and in a flash of inspiration realised that the markings on the shell of the tortoise (which had just inched towards him on to the bank) held the key to the entire universe.

It gets much more complicated after this, and several books are excellent in explaining the intricacies of the philosophy, among them William Spear's *Feng Shui Made Easy*, Sarah Shurety's *Feng Shui*, Phillippa Waring's *The Way of Feng Shui*, as well as her book *The Feng Shui of Gardening*.

Modern theorists call feng shui 'the electricity of nature' because of its central principle, which is that all matter has vibration. This vibration, which the Chinese call chi is an invisible energy which flows constantly through all life forms.

fortune. In every early culture, houses were built near sites of clear water. In classical feng shui the front door would be organised to face water flowing towards or alongside it. However, short of rebuilding your neighbourhood, what can you do to increase the energy and improve the balance in your own home?

You could place a small fountain, a water sculpture or perhaps a bird bath near the entrance to your house. As William Spear notes, make sure these are well maintained, because stagnant water creates 'confusion' and defeats the purpose of activating energy. Inside your house an aquarium creates a 'double' cure, according to Spear, because it 'incorporates both the symbolism of good fortune contained

'Our nature lies in movement; complete calm is death.'

Keeping the pathways of your body and your environment clear allows the free and easy movement of energy. Overall, feng shui illuminates the need for rebalancing your energy naturally.

This involves considerable knowledge and planning of both your inner and outer worlds as well knowing how to forge and maintain a relationship between them. The promised rewards are considerable: prosperity and longevity.

To most Westerners feng shui is simply concerned with the proper placement of objects in the house offering quite logical, obvious suggestions such as 'Don't place your bed in the doorway' and so on. But these are superficial tips of the iceberg, as it were, of the wide-ranging philosophy of feng shui and don't explain how 'the way of wind and water' can energise your environment.

Water is synonymous with life. It is a symbol of good

in the tank and activity expressed by the live fish'. (Now you know why every Chinese restaurant has an aquarium as you enter.) Whatever water element you decide on, do not put it in the north-east corner of your home. This is not good feng shui.

Moving water can have a beneficial effect. French philosopher Pascal underlines the importance of movement itself: 'Our nature lies in movement; complete calm is death.' You only need to look at the quickening of life by water to understand the relationship of water to life. Movement is an expression of energy and water epitomises that energy. Outside, should you live in a house with a garden, you want to surround the house with energy. This comes from plants and water. Sarah Surety comments that 'if you are lucky, you will have a stream that is flowing eastward'. She emphasises that water is 'the life blood of a garden as it cleanses and revitalises the immediate area and improves your luck'. The contrast between textures is important, so if you have a pond, it is pleasing to have a rockery nearby. For inspiration, read Anthony Archer-Wills' latest book, *Water Power*.

VISIT MONET'S LANDSCAPE OF REFLECTION

The French Impressionist Claude Monet is probably best known for his paintings of the water lilies in his garden at Giverny. That magical place became his life and in inspiring him it has inspired millions, not only from visiting it, but also through his paintings.

The garden at Giverny is open every day except Monday from April to November, so give yourself a day off, jump in the car with a friend and shuttle over to see it – it's an easy drive

provides a direct reference to something inside yourself. The very rhythm of day and night, of the moon, the tides, the seasons, of the weather on a single day can feed or deplete your soul, and it is all too easy to ignore or lose track of these rhythms, especially if you live in a city.

If you are thinking, 'But I don't much like the country' or 'I am not a "nature" person', you may be misreading how the outer and inner worlds connect. As a result, you could be starving your body and soul; closing yourself off from a more satisfying, productive life. According to Novalis, the great eighteenth-century German poet: 'The seat of the soul is there where the inner and outer worlds meet.'

That is why it is important to become open to the weather. I mean this literally and metaphorically. When we moved to

Nature is many things, but above all it provides a direct reference to something inside yourself.

from Calais. Tel: 00332 3251 2821. For armchair travellers, there is also an excellent video of Monet's Giverny Gardens by TwoFour Productions, the team responsible for the BBC2 television series. It took a year to make, follows the full cycle of the garden and explores the relationship between Monet's garden and his art. To order (£14.99) and for information ring: + 44 (0) 1752 345424. Their website offers a list of gardening videos: www.twofour.co.uk.

BECOME 'OPEN TO THE WEATHER'

As a writer, I find it essential to water my soul with natural and man-made sources in the environment, as well as with painting and poetry. Shakespeare said that art is a mirror held up to nature. Nature is many things, but above all it

Cornwall, I became interested in the Newlyn group of painters who, at the turn of the last century, took their brushes and easels outside to paint *en plein air*. This was not a new idea. The French were already out there painting away on the opposite shore in Brittany. The idea was to release the painter from the confines of the studio to sense nature in the raw.

For me, the principle of *en plein air* painting brought to life the concept that you have to be open to the weather in order to connect with nature, to replenish your spirit and water your soul. The British painter, John Birch, spent his life by water, painting and fishing all day in a secluded, idyllic cove called Lamorna, just west of Penzance in Cornwall. He gave himself the middle name Lamorna to distinguish himself from another painter called John Birch, but my rather romantic notion is that he was so taken with the place that he took its name. His work inspired this poem, which I wrote after many great walks on the rugged Cornish coast:

En Plein Air
i.m. Samuel Johnson Lamorna Birch, 1869–1955

He stands, open to the weather,
mixing colours, mimicking gulls,
drinking in the oceanic light.
Like a captain, he eyes the sea,
allowing the winds to guide his elbow. They take him

well out of his depth. *This is like drowning....*
He stabs at the air – he gets a rush
stronger than the incoming tide. Onto that dry

sandy stretch, wave follows wave, foam-flecked,
uncurling from his loaded brush. *It's a start.*

The name of this place will become his own:
the Anglo-Saxon tall-masted Birch,
prefaced with a steepled Celtic Cove. For sixty years
he'll fish the river and work the sea, capturing waves,
letting them go. Barehanded, his last words will be...

'how I would paint...'

Listen to your instinct. It will lead you to a place that makes you feel whole. It might even be your own house or garden where a pond, a simple fountain – indoors or out – or just a simple terracotta pot that fills with rain (and a diving frog) will provide the sight, sound and energy of moving water.

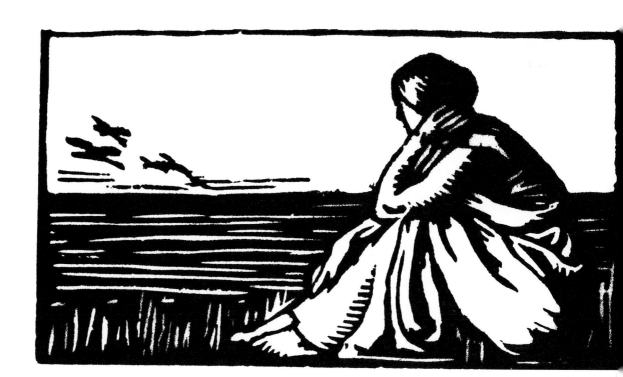

Right:
The Marsh, woodcut
by Gwen Raverat.

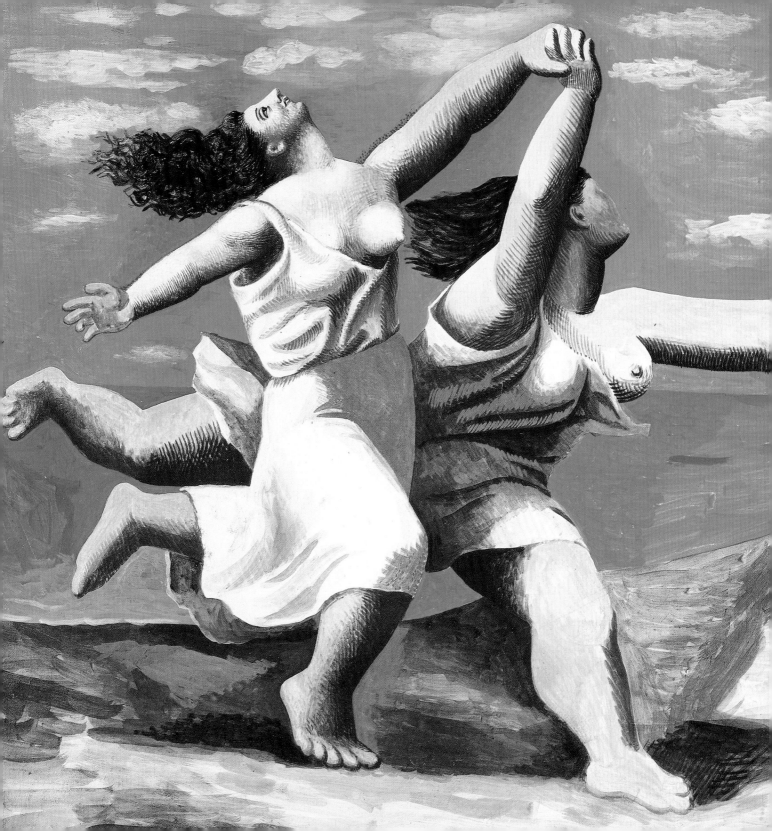

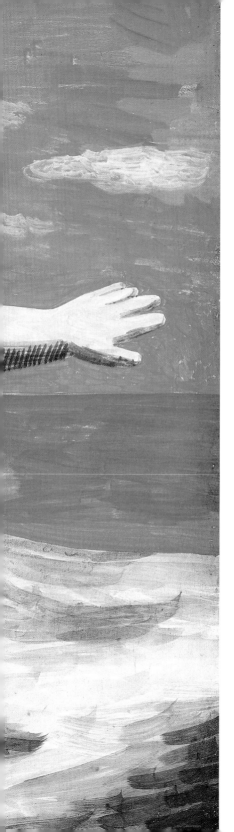

'Water is the one substance from which the earth can conceal nothing. It sucks out its innermost secrets and brings them to our very lips.

JEAN CHIRADOUX
THE MADWOMAN OF CHAILLOT

Two women running on the beach or The race, 1922 by Pablo Picasso

directory

SPAS

St David's Hotel and Spa
Havannah Street, Cardiff Bay, CF10 5SD. Tel: +44 (0)2920 454045. Website: www.spaview.com. *Day and residential spa. Facilities include hydrotherapy bath and pool, 'sanarium' and gym.*

The Balmoral Health Club, Balmoral Hotel
1 Princes Street, Edinburgh, EH2 2EQ. Tel: +44 (0)131 622 8880. *Day spa. Includes gym, pool and steam room.*

The Club at County Hall
Westminster Bridge Road, London, SE1 7PB. Tel: +44 (0)20 7928 4900. *Facilities include swimming pool, Jacuzzi, gym, and steam, sauna and relaxation rooms. Day packages available.*

The Berkeley Health Club and Spa
Wilton Place, Knightsbridge, London, SW18 7RL. Tel: +44 (0)20 7235 6000. Website: www.savoy-group.co.uk. *Day spa. Gym, sauna, stream room and pool. Facials, body scrubs and other treatments available.*

Dorchester Hotel
Park Lane, London, W1A 2HJ. Tel: +44 (0)20 7495 7335 *Day spa. Offers range of hydrotherapy treatments, including hydrotherapy bath and contrast showers.*

Champneys Piccadilly
21a Piccadilly, London, W1 0VH. Tel: +44 (0)20 7255 8000. Website: www.champneys.com. *Swimming pool, Jacuzzi, and eight treatment rooms offering over 70 therapies.*

Claridges, Olympus Suite
Brook Street, Mayfair, London W1A 2JQ. Tel: +44 (0)20 7629

8860. *Small peaceful spa/gym offering various seaweed and mud-based treatments.*

Depilex Health Studios
71 Welbeck Street, London. Tel: +44 (0)20 7486 0852. *Offers seaweed-based body wraps, facials and products.*

The Grove
182–4 Kensington Church Street, London, W8 4DP. Tel: +44 (0)20 7221 2266. *Spa and gym includes a complementary health clinic for a total holistic approach.*

Harrods Ladies Hair and Beauty Salon
Knightsbridge, London, SW1X 7XL, London. Tel: +44 (0)20 7893 8333. *Seaweed scrubs, body wraps, massages.*

Aveda Concept Salon
at Harvey Nichols. 109–125 Knightsbridge, London, SW1X 7RJ. Tel: +44 (0)20 7235 5000. *Treatments include the Hydrotherm Massage and seaweed wraps.*

Aveda's Urban Retreat
at Harvey Nichols. 107-11 Briggate LS1 6AZ, Leeds. Tel: +44 (0)113 204 8888. *Offers a day-long total experience of various treatments.*

Livingwell Clubs.
Tel 0800 136 6363 for your nearest club. *Health clubs across Britain.*

Tyringham Naturopathic Clinic
Tyringham, Newport Pagnell, MK16 9ER. Tel +44 (0)1908 610450. *Rigorous treatments.*

INTERNATIONAL SPAS

The Soho Sanctuary
119 Mercer, between Prince Street and Spring Street, New York. Tel: 00 1 212-334-5550. *Beauty and relaxation achieved through massage and mud therapy.*

BlissOut
568 Broadway and 57, 19 East 57th Street, New York.

Tel: +1 212 219 8970. Website: www.blissworld.com. *Day spa. Treatments include facials and hydrotherapy baths.*

The Repêchage Spa
115 East 57th Street, New York, New York. Tel: +1 212 319 1770. *Thalassotherapy treaments.*

Aida Thibiant European Day Spa
499 N. Canon Drive, Beverly Hills, Los Angeles, California. Tel: 00 1 (310) 278-7565. *Individual treatments or day packages including the patented Hydromassage Shower.*

The Lodge Spa
Inchydoney Island, Co. Cork, Eire. Tel: +353 (0)233 3143. *Luxurious residential spa. Thalassotherapy treatments.*

Villa Thalgo
218 rue du Faubourg St-Honoré, Paris. Tel: 0033 1 45 62 00 20 *Day spa offering thalassotherapy treatments in urban setting.*

The Relaxation Centre at the Hotel Capital
111 Darlinghust Road, Sydney. Tel: 0061 (0)2-9358-2755. *Rigorous hydrotherapy and massage treatments.*

Domaine du Royal Club Evian at the Hotel Royal,
74500, Evian, France. Tel: 00 33 45026 8500. *Wide range of expertly delivered hydrotherapy and massage methods in luxurious setting.*

Chiva-Som International Health Resort,
73/4 Petchkasem Rd, Hua Hin, 7110 Thailand. Tel: 00 66 32 5536 536 or Seasons in Style on 0151 342-0505. *The ultimate spa experience.*

Thalassa Quiberon
Pointe de Goulvars Brittany, France Telephone Erna Low for all bookings: + 44 (0) 270 584-2841. *Thalassotherapy carried out under medical supervision.*

Ojo Caliente Mineral Springs Resort
Ojo Caliente, New Mexico, USA. Tel: 00 1 800-222-9162. *The oldest health spa in North America.*

SPA BOOKING AND INFORMATION
Erna Low
Tel: +44 (0)20 7584 2841. *Specialises in arranging tailor-made residential spa holidays outside the UK.*

Healthy Venues
Tel: 024 7669 0300. Website: www.healthyvenues.co.uk. *They represent and take bookings for many spas throughout the United Kingdom.*

Spa Reine
Office du Tourism, Place Royale 41, 4900 Spa, Belgium. Tel: (32) 87 79 53 53. Fax: (32) 77 79 53 54. *The historic spa town offers many different treatments.*

BEAUTY PRODUCTS AND TREATMENTS
BlissOut
Tel: +1 888 243 8825 for mail-order catalogue. Website: www.blissworld.com *Wide range of marine based products.*

Droyt's
Progress Mill, Chorley PR6 0RZ. Tel: +44 (0)1257 417251. email: sales@droyts.com. *Wide range of beautiful soaps and bath products.*

Kobashi
2 Fore Street, Ide, Devon, EX2 9RQ. Tel: +44 (0)1392 217628. Website: www.kobashi.com. *Suppliers of pure essential oils.*

Lush
Tel: +44 (0)1202 668545 or see www.lush.co.uk for mail order or your nearest shop. *Fresh and handmade cosmetics.*

Thalgo
Tel 0800 146041 or see www.thalgo.com. *World leaders in marine skin care products.*

Repêchage
Tel 0800 731 7546 for UK stockists. Website: www.repechage.com. Mail order available. *Specialise in seaweed-based products.*

E'spa
Tel +44 (0)1252 741600 for UK stockists. *Essential oils, and products based on them.*

Elemis
Tel: +44 (0)20 8954 8033 for stockists and mail-order. *For good body brushes.*

The Body Shop
Tel: 01903 731 500 for your nearest branch. Website: www.the-body-shop.com. *Excellent source of bath and shower treats, terrific body brushes, aromatherapy candles, lotions and potions.*

Algascience
Tel: +44 (0)1488 648319 for stockists. *Seaweed-based cosmetics and treatments.*

Erno Laszlo.
Tel: +44 (0)345 697072 for mail order details. *Range of soaps and beauty products.*

BATHROOMS
Alison White
Tel +44 (0) 270 609-6127. Website: www.alisonwhiteblinds.com *Imaginative and original window blinds.*

Aston-Matthews
141–47 Essex Road, Islington N1 2SN. Tel: + 44 (0)20 7226 7220. *Wide range of bathroom hardware.*

Lyn Le Grice
Tel +44 (0)1736 364 193 for information, or to arrange a consultation. *For ideas on creating your spa/bathroom.*

Ocean
Tel: 0870 84 84 84 0 for mail-order catalogue. *Beautiful bathroom hardware.*

The White Company
Tel +44 (0)20 7385-7988 for mail order. *Beautiful white 100 per cent cotton towels, plus simple bath mats and bathrobes. Despite their name, they do towels in colours, too.*

SWIMMING
Pierre Gruneberg
For a video of his method (£13) ring +44 (0)20 7413 9582. To contact him in summer: Club Dauphin, Grand Hôtel, Cap Ferrat. Tel: +33 4 93 765 050; fax: +33 4 93 761 397. To find out where in America he teaches, contact him in France.
In Britain, he teaches at the following two hotels which offer group or individual classes at different times of the year: The Runnymede Hotel and Spa, Surrey (tel: + 44 (0)1784 436171) and Hollington House Hotel, near Newbury, Wiltshire (tel: + 44 (0) 1635-255100).

Shaw Method of Swimming
Tel +44 (0)20 8446 9442 or +44 (0)20 8445-8693. Website: www.@art-of-swimming.com.

Feng Shui UK
Tel/Fax: +44 (0)1373 474085. *For advice on using the power of water in your home and garden.*

Vessel
114 Kensington Park Road, W11 2PW. Tel: +44 (0)20 7727 8001. *For beautiful drinking glasses, jugs and carafes.*

bibliography

WATERING YOUR BODY

British Dietetic Association, Elizabeth House, 22 Suffolk Street, Queensway, Birmingham B1 1LS (Send a sae for a free copy of *Fabulous Food Facts*)

Chaitow, Leon *Hydrotherapy*, Element Books Limited 1999

Clarke, Jane *Body Foods for Life*, Weidenfeld and Nicolson 1999

Deakin, Roger *Waterlog*, Chatto & Windus 1999

Fox, R Fortescue MD (intro.) *The Spas of Britain*, The Pitman Press, Bath n.d._

Herbert, Arthur Stanley *The Hot Springs of New Zealand*, H.K. Lewis & Co. 1921

Hembry, Phyllis *British Spas from 1815 to the Present*, The Athlone Press 1997

Hodgkinson, Liz *The Drinking Water Cure*, Carnell plc 1996

Holford, Patrick *The Optimum Nutrition Bible*, Piatkus 1999

Johnson, James M.D. *Pilgrimages to the Spas*, London: S. Highley 1841

Kenton, Leslie *10 Steps to a New You*, Ebury Press 1999

Kenton, Leslie *Passage to Power*, Vermilion 1998

Le Grice, Lyn *The Art of Stencilling*, Penguin 1986

McCloud, Kevin *The Complete Decorator*, Ebury Press 1996

Muryn, Mary *Water Magic: Healing Bath Recipes*, Bantam 1997

Neville Havins, Peter J. *The Spas of England*, Robert Hale & Company 1976

Northrup, Dr Christiane *Women's Bodies Women's Wisdom*, BCA 1998

Porter, Roy *The Greatest Benefit to Mankind*, Harper Collins 1997

Rae, W. Fraser *Austrian Health Resorts*, Chapman and Hall Ltd. 1889

Silver, Helene *Rejuvenate: A 21-Day Natural Detox Plan for Optimal Health*, The Crossing Press, California, 1998

Schauberger, Viktor *The Water Wizard*, Gateway Books 1998

Wilson, Erasmus *The Eastern, or Turkish Bath*, John Churchill 1861

Wyllie, Timothy *Dolphins Telepathy & Underwater Birthing*, Bear & Co Inc. 1993

WATERING YOUR SOUL

Archer-Wills, Anthony *Water power: A Unique Approach to Designing Water Gardens*, Conran Octopus 1999

Arnoux, Jean-Claude *The Ultimate Water Garden Book*, Batsford 1996

Bartlett, Jennifer *In the Garden*, Harry N. Abrams, Inc. 1982

Bord, Janet and Colin *Sacred Waters*, Granada 1985

Campbell, Joseph *The Hero with a Thousand Faces*, Fontana Press 1993

Coleman, Simon & Elsner, John *Pilgrimage*, British Museum Press 1995

Davies, Vivian and Friedman, Renée *Egypt*, British Museum Press 1998

Frazer, Sir James *The Golden Bough*, Wordsworth Editions Ltd 1993

Greene, Liz *Astrology for Lovers*, Thorsons 1999

Greene, Liz *The Astrology of Fate*, George Allen & Unwin 1984

Harvey, Charles and Suzi *Principles of Astrology*, Thorsons 1999

Leakey, Richard & Lewin, Roger *People of the Lake*, Collins 1979

Meyrick, J. *Holy Wells*, Published by J. Meyrick 1982

Michell, John *Sacred England*, Gothic Image Publications 1996

Porter, Eliot, and Levi, Peter *The Greek World*, Aurum Press 1981

Quiller-Couch, Arthur (editor) *The Oxford Book of English Verse*, OUP 1916

Shurety, Sarah *Feng Shui For Your Home*, Ebury Press 1997

Soothill, Eric and Thomas, Michael J. *The Natural History of Britain's Coasts*, Blandford Press, 1988

Skafte, Dianne *When Oracles Speak*, Thorsons 1997

Walker, Barbara G. *The Woman's Encyclopedia of Myths and Secrets*, Harper & Row 1983

Waring, Philippa *The Feng Shui of Gardening*, Souvenir Press 1998

index

The Publisher would like to thank the
following for the kind permission to
reproduce the following excerpts:

Excerpt from *'Dinner with Persephone'*
by Patricia Storace reproduced with the
permission of Granta Books, London
and Pantheon Books, New York.

Excerpt from Jo Shapcott's *'In the Bath'*
reproduced with the kind permission of
Faber and Faber Ltd.

'Seascape' from THE COMPLETE
POEMS 1927–1979 by Elizabeth Bishop.
Copyright © 1979, 1983 by Alice Helen
Methfessel. Reprinted by permission of
Farrar, Straus and Giroux, LLC.

acknowledgments

The author would like to thank Jane Turnbull, my agent, for her initial enthusiasm for this project, for her creative advice and unfailing support throughout the process. I would also like to thank Sara Ann Freed who sparked to this idea from the very start, for her encouragement throughout, and for her helpful contributions to the spa section.

I am very grateful to Charles Thomas for allowing me to reproduce his precious drawing; also for sourcing and lending me precisely the books I needed from his private library. My thanks also to Melissa Hardie for her generous loan of so many relevant books from the invaluable Hypatia Library.

I have been greatly helped by Jessica Mann's expert guidance on the complicated issues and aspects concerning the purity of water. I would like to thank Di Downs whose fluent French helped me to begin my research on thalassotherapy. Christine Graham-Vivian was unstinting in her time and effort to educate me on garden history and design, as was Anne Wickett on the philosophy of Feng Shui. Elisabeth Constantine gave valuable suggestions regarding the energetic qualities of water. Tim Hosken, homeopathic vet, was instrumental in explaining the process of cellular osmosis. Many thanks to them all.

I am extremely grateful to Jo Shapcott for allowing me to reprint a portion of her wonderful poem. My thanks, also, to Mike Murphy for taking the trouble to lead me to Thoreau's ideal quotation on water.

My thanks to Jane Turnbull, Michelle, and Rachael Pearson for their lively and informative first person accounts which bring to life those sections of the book in which they appear. I would like to thank John Simeoni for his imaginative and inspiring conceptual ideas at the start of the project, and to Val Simeoni for all her exacting work in implementing them.

My husband Fred Taylor has been my mainstay throughout the journey of this book. It would not have been possible to complete it in the time given without his dedicated input as historian and researcher.

The Publisher would like to thank the following people and organisations for permission to reproduce the photographs listed below.

2 The National Mineral Water Information Service; **3** Pamela Hanson © Vogue/The Condé Nast Publications Limited; **5** Colorific; **6** The Dorchester Spa; **8–9** Telegraph Colour Library; **10–11** John Simeoni; **16–17 & 23** Gettyone Stone; **18–19** Vessel; **28** © The British Museum; **29** Telegraph Colour Library; **35** Vessel; **38–9** Images Colour Library, **44–5** Vessel; **46–7** Telegraph Colour Library; **49** Superstock; **50** Telegraph Colour Library; **51** *top left* Telegraph Colour Library; **54–5 & 142–3** Telegraph Colour Library; **65** Clay Perry; **66** Barbara and Zafer Baran/Special Photographers Library; **72 & 72–3** The White Company; **73** *top right* Mike Greenslade; **77** The Dorchester Spa; **84** Telegraph Colour Library; **88** The Dorchester Spa; **104** Telegraph Colour Library; **112** Telegraph Colour Library; **114–15** Telegraph Colour Library; **119** Gettyone Stone; **120–1** Alice Kavounas; **125** Strigils and sponges, 1879 (proof engraving) by Sir Lawrence Alma-Tadema (1836–1912), British Museum, London, UK/Bridgeman Art Library; **126** Alice Kavounas; **131** Charles Thomas **135** Mick Sharp Library; **136–37** Grant V Faint/ The Image Bank; **139** Mike Greenslade; **141** Telegraph Colour Library; **145** Gettyone Stone; **146** Mike Greenslade; **149** © The Marsh, Estate of Gwen Raverat, 2000; **150–1** Two women running on the beach or the race, 1922 (gouache on plywood) by Pablo Picasso (1881–1973) Museé Picasso, Paris, France/Peter Willi/Bridgeman Art Library © Succession Picasso/DACS 2000